FOREWORD BY DR. MICHELE WELLS PHD, MSW

FROM THE DEPTH OF MY SOUL

MY JOURNEY OUT OF DEPRESSION

LICHELLE L. BEELER

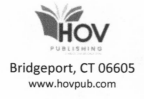

Bridgeport, CT 06605
www.hovpub.com

From the Depth of My Soul:
My Journey out of Depression

HOV Publishing a division of HOV, LLC.
Bridgeport, CT 06605
Email: hopeofvision@gmail.com
www.hovpub.com

Cover Design: Hope of Vision Designs
Editor: Sonya Peters Bailey

Contact the Author, Lichelle L. Beeler at: beelerlichelle262@yahoo.com

For further information regarding special discounts on bulk purchases, please visit www.hovpub.com or contact hopeofvision@gmail.com.

ISBN Paperback: 978-1-955107-67-9
ISBN eBook: 978-1-955107-66-2

Printed in the United States of America

DEDICATION

I dedicate this book to my parents. To my father, who encouraged me in writing at an early age and who nurtured that creative gift in me to tell stories, never knowing that I would one day explore and share my own story. Dadoo, I am fighting to overcome a battle that you were not afforded to win against depression. When I think about giving up, I think about how I would be destroying your legacy. And so, I continue to fight, and I will continue to fight for us. To my mother, an angel appeared to me about five months after you died to deliver a message to me. The message was that you were having trouble adjusting to being on the other side because of your worries for me. The angel told me that you were aware that I had the tendency to go to this dark place. Mommy, I hope that you see me now gaining victory over what imprisoned me for many years, and I pray that you are resting now knowing that I am well. I still live for you. I would never want to grieve you, not even in death. I will be all that you both hoped I would be. Thank you for being my parents and for loving me. I love you both, from the depth of my soul.

ACKNOWLEDGEMENTS

To my Heavenly Father. I thank You for giving me the wisdom and fortitude to finish this assignment. Without You I am and can do nothing, but with You I can do all things; for You give me strength. I know that as long as I depend on You that my steps will be ordered to have great success. And, as long as I live, I will always love and follow after You.

To my brother, Mark. Thank you for being not only my brother but for also being my protector, my greatest support, and my friend. I will forever be grateful to you for giving me the space I needed to heal. Mama said that one day we would only have each other, and I have found that to be true. I would not want to do life without you.

To my dearest friend and sissy, Dr. Michele. You have been the glue that has held me together when it seemed that everything in me was falling apart. Your love and faith in me gave me the hope I needed to continue on my journey. You are one of the best things that has ever happened to me. I can never repay you, but I will spend the rest of my life trying.

To my friend and seester, Natasha. You truly are my "ride or die". Your prayers backed the enemy up off of me when the battle became too much. You understand me. You don't judge me, but you tell me the truth, and you hold me accountable to what you know is in me. Thank you for being my friend when I did not deserve it. You taught me the true power of forgiveness and restoration. You taught me that no matter what it may look like, I can begin again.

To Pastor Nina Anderson and the Well Ministry. Thank you for being a bridge over troubled water. Your ministry lifted me when nothing else seemed to help. You taught me to dig deeper and to develop a passion for God's Word and for His ways in ways I had never experienced before. I will forever be thankful for your ministry, and whenever you need me, I will do my absolute best to be there for you as you were for me.

To my special sorority sisters and sands, Deiona "Dede", Luretia "Dany", and Ursula. Thank you for your unconditional love. Thank you for the daily check-ins. Thank you for the weekend getaways. Thank you for your compassion and understanding and for teaching me the value of true sisterhood. I only pray to be the same support to you as you have been to me.

To my dear and special cousins, Kelli, Angela, and (Auntie/Mom) Emma. Thank you for allowing me to experience family again. I didn't know how much I needed you, but I certainly did. You have all been an extension of my mother's love to me. I am proud and blessed to call you my family.

To my friend and sister, Kelli. Thank you for being such a loyal friend and thank you for reconnecting me with being back home. You are one of the kindest persons I have ever experienced. I appreciate you spending time with me and you listening to me when I truly needed an ear. I love you girl.

To my friend and sister, Carmen. Thank you for your friendship. Even when I isolated and you did not hear from me, I knew you were aware of my struggle and that you were praying for me. Thank you for allowing me to be more than a friend but to be your sister. I hope I am able to make you proud seeing me STAND again.

To my friend and sissy, Sheryl. Thank you for being there when I needed to have the tough conversations. Thank you for convincing me to put my mental health first. Even in your own struggles, you still lift me up, and you make me believe that my friendship makes a difference. I am so glad we got into that fight in high school because it blossomed into a beautiful friendship and sisterhood. I love you so much.

To my friend, Mary "Goobie". You were the first person who made me feel welcome in returning to live back home. You always invited me and included me in things. Being in your wedding was one of my greatest joys because you shared such an intimate moment of your life with me, and I thank you for that. Thank you for continuing to invite me to things even when I would not accept. I asked you not to give up on me, and you did not. You are forever etched into my heart.

To my friend and sister, Terrie. I will cherish you always. You were one of the few people in Fort Wayne who saw my pain and tried to help me. I want you to know that your labor has not been in vain and that I have not, nor will I ever forget you and what you did for me. Thank you for praying me through many dark days. I share this reward with you.

To my friend and dear sister, Jamiene "Mimi". When no one else was there, you became my prayer partner, and your prayers helped me through a very difficult season in my life. I pray that you know how pivotal your love was to me. I would not have survived that season without you. I thank you for that and for your continued friendship.

To my dear friend, Trico, who is now resting in Heaven. I wish I could have had the opportunity to tell you how much I appreciated you. You brought life and laughter into my home, and you helped me to not feel so alone. I tried to give you back a portion of what you had given me. You were a true and loyal friend to the end. I miss you so much. I will love you forever.

To my friend, Gary Jr. From the bottom of my heart, thank you for the support you provided to me in your own special way. I will never forget.

To Dr. Kevin Cosby, Sr., Pastor of St. Stephen Baptist Church. Your teaching has been critical to my livelihood. I am so grateful for the tools you have provided to help me stand strong in the Lord. Truly you have been and are a blessing to my life. Coming to church and tuning into the messages every week changed and saved my life.

To Professor Lori Paris. Thank you for your understanding and for your support while I was your student and even beyond that. You believed in me when I no longer believed in myself, and you gave me the help I needed during such a challenging time in my life. I wish that every professor was like you. I am so glad to have met you. I only hope to be as effective as the type of clinician in which you are. I will always view you as my mentor and strive to follow your example.

To my former principal, Kim Morales. Thank you for being who you are. You went above and beyond the call of duty to express your concern and to demonstrate your support for me. Thank you for sitting down with me and striving to understand. Thank you for not making me feel bad for putting my mental health before my position. There are not many bosses like you. I am glad to have worked with you and to have experienced you in that way. You are the best.

To the doctors and therapists that have worked with me. I am thankful for your patience and for your support. I am especially thankful to my primary care physician, Dr. Robert Johnson, who has worked tirelessly with me to help me find the right combination of medication, vitamins, and healthy life habits that would allow me to live the best life possible. I appreciate you for answering every question, for explaining things, and for encouraging me when I was discouraged. You have played an enormous role in my healing process.

Finally, I want to thank every person who has ever called my name out in prayer and who has ever offered a word of encouragement to me. I used to believe in a philosophy which said that being alone makes you strong. I no longer believe that; I now believe that being alone does not make you strong but that it makes you weak and vulnerable. I realize now that I cannot do this alone and that I need the help of every person I can get in order to make it on this journey. I am so thankful for you all. Please do not stop praying for me. I love you, and I need you to survive.

CONTENTS

FOREWORD

Dr. Michele Wells PhD, MSW

The Depth of My Soul: My Journey out of Depression is an intensely honest and real look at living life with clinical depression. The life that many are living, but are afraid to expose because of how they will be viewed by others. In our encounters with people we often see the end result without knowing the many valleys that were walked through to get to the person that is presented before us. From The Depth of My Soul: My Journey out of Depression is a journey to health and wholeness that comes through the deep dark waters of depression. Lichelle has allowed herself to be vulnerable about the wounds, hurts, and pain that wanted to take her out of this world. She has opened the door to the depth of the darkness and revealed that there is a light at the end of it. Psalm 139:12 says it well of our Lord, "but even in darkness I cannot hide from you. To you the night shines as bright as day. Darkness and light are the same to you." In the midst of the darkness the light of the Lord in Lichelle guided her back from depression as He took each step with her to her final destination…freedom. In His presence she is now experiencing how the Lord wants to use her for those of us who need a roadmap to navigate either walking through depression personally or loving someone that is in its clutches.

The journey has not been easy! I wondered many times, was I going to lose my friend to this darkness. Loved ones often do not understand the journey, so they just expect the person to get over it or just be happy. This book is evidence that clinical depression, like any other physical illness, needs treatment. The person needs the support of loved ones, not their judgement. Lichelle fought through the stigma that the world places on mental illness. Lichelle stood up against the answer that so many give when they do not want to deal with the truth of this illness… "just pray about it." This response minimizes the tools that are provided by the Lord (the skill of a therapist or the use of medication). People respond in this way because we do not want to deal with what we don't understand. Lichelle, in her fight, brings understanding that ALL of what the Lord has provided through the knowledge and gifting of men can be used to bring healing and restoration. Lichelle is an educator that has educated herself and others on the many facets of depression. Lichelle is an advocate that understands and stands for those that need to be free of the stigma of mental illness and given permission to use what is available to them to begin their journey out of depression toward freedom. Lichelle is an expert. Her experience is her expertise! From The Depth of My Soul: My Journey out of Depression is a guide for you and I in how we move forward in loving and supporting those with depression. It is a look at the scars that can contribute to someone not making it out of depression. It is a look into Lichelle's life that gives the reader a greater depth of understanding in how to help and not hinder. It is a journey of a life that honors the Lord through vulnerability and strength simultaneously.

From The Depth of My Soul: My Journey out of Depression needs to be in the hands of anyone who has ever dealt with or loved someone with mental illness. Lichelle's work lets us know that there is a way forward through the love of Christ and the love of others who would offer support for the journey! Embrace this work and share it so that we can be better for one another on the road to complete health and wholeness.

CHAPTER 1

Introduction

I'm lying in a bed in a hotel room. I have nowhere to go. I have been living with my brother for the past few months. My brother. My brother who I thought wanted me with him. My brother who I thought was my protector and who would never do anything to hurt me. And yet, I am lying here with my heart crushed into a million pieces, and I have no idea if it can ever be repaired. I call two people to inform them of what is going on and my whereabouts, my therapist and my very good friend and sister, Michele. I had only been with this new therapist for a short while. I had been seeing a therapist virtually, through the local seminary for several months during the pandemic. However, we ended our relationship. My therapist was an MAFT student, and she was graduating. Besides, she felt I needed more support from a licensed clinical social worker. For whatever reason, I felt comfortable with calling my new therapist. In fact, I felt I had to in order to keep myself from doing something I would later regret. I had no idea what to do. The only other person who knew what I had been going through completely was Michele. She and I had been close for many years. We are like David and Jonathan in the Bible. Because she prays and intercedes with me regularly, I believe God shows her things about me without me having to share them. She knows when I am going through things. I am able to freely share with her and be honest with her without judgment, and she always meets me with compassion, grace, and love.

Michele was the only other person I told that I had left my brother's house in the middle of the night ready to end it all. On this night, I felt the lowest and loneliest I had ever felt in my entire life. My mother was gone. My father was not mentally well. My family was distant and divided. My close friends were not there. Many had no idea what I was going through. Some, I wondered if they even cared. Some were going through their own challenges as well during the pandemic. For the past almost year, I had isolated myself from everything and everyone. I did not go anywhere or do anything. It really was not noticed because of the pandemic, no one was doing much of anything or going anywhere. We had all been sheltered inside of our homes. A few months before I ended up here, my brother had moved into his new home. He went through a divorce the previous year and was rebuilding his life. He stayed with me in my one-bedroom apartment for a few months, but he found his own home quickly. I was not working and had no income. I was fortunate to have a large savings. I had been saving to purchase my own home. I had been without a car payment for quite some time. There had also been a stop put on student loan payments during the pandemic. So, this helped a lot. I had every intention of just staying in my apartment in order to not become a burden to my brother. However, he suggested I move with him in order to not go through all of my savings and to focus on returning back to work. I had been off work since the start of the school year.

When the pandemic hit, school was closed, and learning became virtual. Those were the worst two months of my teaching career ever. I struggled to get out of bed to attend meetings, compile lessons, make assignments, assess learning, contact parents, and everything else required of me all virtually. To be honest, I did very little, not even the minimum. I was thankful for the year to finally be over and thought I would take the summer to get better and be ready to return to work in the fall. However, when the fall came, that did not happen at all. Staff was to return to work about three days before students. I had been so out of the loop. I was not checking emails or anything that summer. I had no idea of when school actually started. That entire summer, I was in bed. My routine was the same pretty much every day. I slept all day, stayed up all night, and ate terribly. I gained an enormous amount of weight. My apartment was a mess. It became so bad that I had gnats everywhere, and I did not even care. I was not washing my dishes or clothes or emptying the trash, and my personal hygiene was nonexistent. My brother did come help me clean and to get rid of the gnats. It was extremely embarrassing, but I could not have done it on my own, and I would not have allowed anyone else to visit. Even after cleaning everything, there was a pile of clothes that sat on my bed. I could not tell what was clean or dirty, and the thought of me going through them to find out and to wash them and fold or hang them was so overwhelming I could not do it. So, they just remained on one side of my bed while I slept on the other side. Eventually, when my brother came to stay with me, I put them in garbage bags and just put them in my bedroom closet, out of sight and out of mind. I think I finally just threw the bags of clothes away and aimed to start over. Michele had advised me that if I had not worn them in all of this time and if it was going to make me feel worse to just get rid of them, and I am glad I did.

Moving to my brother's was very difficult for me. While he was at work, I desperately tried to have the energy to pack up my things. I was moving very slowly, and my brother had to get on my case often. I was trying to be somewhat organized because I knew that if I was not that it was going to cause me even more stress when I had to unpack things. We threw away my bed because it was not usable, and I bought a new bed. My brother quickly set up my bedroom and a small den for me in the third bedroom. I tried to be helpful and buy him a few things that he needed, such as dishes, cookware, and towels and washcloths. I was very happy for my brother. He had been through a lot in his marriage, and I wanted him to be happy. He tried to be helpful to me, but I am sure it was difficult while he was going through his own situation. He worked second shift, so we would sit up at night and watch different TV shows. During the day while he worked, however, I slept. He would encourage me to do certain things, such as take a walk, but I just could not, and I could not explain it to him either. I was severely depressed. It had never gotten this bad before, and I did not know how I was going to survive this time. When I moved into his house, I immediately felt a change. His attitude shifted. It was as though he asked me to be there only because he thought it was the right thing to do but not what he really wanted. He started seeing another woman, and I really felt like I was in the way. I tried to stay in my room and out of the way as much as possible. I bought my own food which was mostly bought fast food or food that I could cook in the microwave because I did not want to use his stove or oven. I did not want to use anything of his. I felt like I was always doing something wrong, even when I tried not to. My brother did not hesitate to let me know. On this particular night, one of the kitchen cabinet doors had fallen off of the hinges when I opened it, and I knew that would be the end of the world. I tried to decide the best time to tell him what had happened, but I knew that no matter what, it was going to be bad. I did not want to text him at work because that would make him angry or tell him as soon as he came home. I had not seen this attitude or side of him when he was staying with me, but all of a sudden, there it was. He really did not want me there. He did not have to say it. I felt it, and

I knew. He discovered the broken cabinet on his own, and he came to my room. I got up to explain it to him and to demonstrate what happened. He was furious. He made the comment that he was not going to be able to have anything nice, because of me, and for me, that was the final straw. He had already been angry with me for other incidents. He became angry one night when I did not completely turn the bathroom faucet off. I had no idea it had to be turned off a certain way. He became angry with me one day when he had left for work and asked me to turn off the sprinkler on his lawn in about twenty minutes, and I forgot. I had a virtual therapy session that lasted for a few hours, and I simply forgot. He had no idea how hard it was for me to just think these days. I am not sure if he even asked. It seemed as though he blamed me for being depressed, like there was something I was doing or not doing to cause myself to be this way. In the few, short conversations I had with him, I quickly realized he simply did not get it, and I was not sure if he ever would. The way he treated my father was a huge clue. My father had also battled mental illness for many years. My brother was very short and impatient with my father, and I did not like it. I took it very personally because I saw myself in my father and oftentimes, I wondered if I would end up the way he had. Nevertheless, on this particular occasion, I was made to feel that I was intentionally trying to destroy my brother's new home and that everything I did was wrong.

I will never forget what he said, how he acted, or how I felt at that moment. I just knew I could not take it.

A few weeks before, I had stayed at a hotel for the weekend to attend a virtual women's retreat that Michele had invited me to. It had been very helpful. Afterwards, I felt I gained some strength to begin taking steps to get back up again. I had been attending Bible studies and prayer meetings virtually, I was committed to my therapy sessions, I had begun walking the neighborhood a little bit, and I had started a new eating plan to lose weight. I was trying. I tried to communicate my plan to my brother, but for him, it was not enough. He did not understand that in order for me to get up, I would first have to start with my spirituality. God was everything to me, and if anyone was going to help me, it was going to be Him. I strongly believed if I could get my relationship with God back on track that I would be able to find the strength I needed to get my life back on track. It is hard to get someone to understand this who does not understand who God truly is to you and who you are in Him.

On this night, I returned to the same hotel. I did not know how long I was going to stay. My immediate thought was that I would find somewhere else to live because I could not stay with my brother any longer. But I also knew that would be difficult. I had money in my savings, but I could not show any income. The only place I could think of that may accept me without providing proof of income was the place I had just rented and left a few months before. Unfortunately, my apartment had been rented, and they did not have any openings. I had applied for long-term disability with my job, but I did not know whether I would get it, how much it would be or how long it would take to receive it. I was essentially stuck. For now, I would take the next few days to just stay in this hotel room where I could eat, sleep, and cry in private. I did not contact my brother, and he did not contact me. Only Michele and my therapist knew where I was, physically and emotionally. Thank God I at least had them.

CHAPTER 2

How Did I Get Here

How did I get here? I'm not just talking about what caused me to leave my brother's in the middle of the night, but how did I get in this position where I was even able to experience the hurt in which I did from my brother. This was early 2021. But things did not start here. I'm going to share the start of this particular episode, but I will later share some experiences that happened even before then. I had experienced major depressive episodes off and on for several years, particularly after my mother passed in 2014. I had sought treatment and taken medication off and on. In 2017, however, I became more hopeful. The year started out with me creating a vision board, something I had never done. In fact, I have not done another one since. The one I did is still hanging on my wall because I have yet to complete everything I envisioned at the start of that year. I have completed some things, and I am very proud of that, but I decided to just leave it up until everything was fulfilled. 2017 brought many good things. I made a big change in my hairstyle which I still have a version of today. I decided to stop going to a hair stylist and to go to a barber instead. I began to rock a fro hawk, and I loved it. I received so many compliments from men and women. It was less maintenance, and I felt truly free. For several years, I had been wanting to leave my profession as a high school teacher, but I was not quite sure what I wanted to do. Several years back, which I will share about later, I had decided I would focus on getting into full-time ministry and serving as a Pastor. However, those plans did not work out. Now, I was more focused on what I could do that would help blend ministry with my career. I needed something that was purposeful, something that I could be passionate about, and something that would pay for my living expenses. Full-time ministry did not seem to be the answer for that, at least not at this time. I knew I wanted to leave teaching. Teaching was something I had wanted to do ever since I was a little girl. However, I had not made the leap to become a counselor or an administrator, so there was nowhere else for me to go in the profession, except the classroom. At one time, I loved teaching, but I no longer did. It had become a job for me, what I did to earn a living. I was no longer as passionate or as effective. In fact, it was beginning to become a chore for me. It affected my mental health tremendously, but I did not know what else I could do. I would spend hours surfing the internet trying to figure out what else I could do with my degrees. After all, I had degrees in education and communication, theatre arts, and English. I was never able to find anything. It was through my own experience that I began to lean more into the mental health field. I realized the power of therapy and how it benefited my life. But I also saw practices I did not like and how I could do things differently. I had begun to learn more about the different roles I could play and the degrees required to allow me to serve in those capacities.

My initial desire was to obtain a Master of Arts in Marriage and Family Counseling or Therapy. This was due to the therapist I had at that time. That was her background, and she really encouraged me. However, the school I wanted to attend did not offer evening classes. My therapist at the time encouraged me to seek God and have faith He would provide for me while I pursued this degree, but I was not there yet. My other option was to attend a school that did offer evening classes, only, they did not offer the same degree. At the other institution, I would have to pursue a Master of Science in Social Work. To my understanding, the end goal would be the same and I would be able to serve as a clinical therapist and practicing therapist. I would be able to attend classes in the evening and maintain my full-time teaching position, just as I had done when pursuing my first master's degree in Secondary Education. Another benefit was that much of my tuition would be covered because of a grant I would receive through working at a struggling high school. I decided that was the path for me, and earlier in that year, I made a decision to start school in the fall. I prayed and asked God to remove the fear I had of completing the program and to give me the strength I needed. My mission statement would become that I wanted to become the help I never received. At this point, I had, had a few different therapists, tried several different medications, but still had not experienced any lasting breakthroughs. I applied to school and was accepted. I just knew this was God's plan for me. I would go to school, and in three years, I would graduate and begin working toward obtaining my certification and licensing to practice social work as a therapist.

Another great thing about 2017 was the position I had taken with my family, physically and emotionally. During Black History month of that year, my Pastor had done a teaching about putting up fences. It was an excellent message about the purpose and necessity of creating boundaries. He explained how boundaries were necessary to prevent toxicity and unnecessary drama in our lives. I took this to heart. All of my life I had struggled with my older siblings and the havoc they caused not only in my life but in others' lives as well. While my mother was living, it was difficult to completely separate myself from that; although for many years I had tried. At the age of seventeen years old, I moved about two and half hours away to attend college. Upon graduation, I moved an hour further than that, where I was about three and a half hours away, and there I stayed for eleven years. It took a lot to bring me back home. I will share more about that later. It was a major hardship that brought me home, but soon after I returned, I remembered why I had left and stayed gone for fifteen years. I remained home for about three years before I left again. This final time that I returned home was due to my mother's death. I had been living across the country and felt I was too far away from what I perceived to be my support system. It is amazing how quickly we forget about why we left something in the first place, and how quickly we remember once we return. When I returned home in 2015, I felt I had made a terrible decision. My family, meaning my older siblings, were no different than when I grew up and when I left. In fact, they were even worse now because my mother had passed, and they were now depending on me to fulfill her role, even though I was the youngest. So, when my Pastor preached that message about boundaries, I knew it was for me, and I aimed to implement it in my life immediately. I decided I would limit the access my older siblings had to me. I stopped making and returning phone calls. I stopped visiting. I stopped celebrating the holidays with them. I stopped allowing them to disturb my peace. Initially, it was easier to do physically than it was to do emotionally. I would hear my mother's voice telling me that I should not do this, that they were my family and that I should just accept them and love them for who they are and be there for them no matter what. There were other so called family members who would try to make me feel the same. But eventually, I was able to silence those voices and do what I felt was best for me, and I did not care what anyone else did, said, thought, or felt. Things were going well until my sister became ill, and it became apparent to me she was not going to live for very much longer. I did not know exactly what her prognosis was, but I just discerned that things were pretty bad and that they were not going to get better. She had done a lot of damage to her body using drugs and consuming alcohol. She was enduring diabetes, mental illness, and doctors were now introducing the possibility of cancer. She wanted to die, and when someone loses the will to live the way she did, there is not much one can do. My advice to my siblings was to make sure her insurance policy was up-to-date, which they did not do, and to consider hospice care for her so she would not suffer. I did go check on her a few times, but I stepped back significantly because I knew my other older siblings would try to make me responsible for her end-of-life care and planning, and I did not want that at all. When my sister died at the end of that year, it was my plan to stand in the background as my older siblings had done all of their lives, allow them to do everything for once, and just show up to pay my respects. However, they handled things so poorly I decided to step in solely to help my nephew. My mother had raised him. He was not as close to his mother. She had been in prison and on the streets for much of his life. Yet, she was still his mother. I knew he loved her and would want to honor her, so I stepped in to support him. It ended up being a disaster. Things eventually came to a full-blown head. While we were at the viewing of my sister's body, because she was going to be cremated and I wanted my nephew to have one final opportunity to see his mother, my older two brothers brought their ignorance and toxicity along with them. I had a feeling thing were not going to go well and had encouraged my brother Mark to attend with me. I was closest to Mark. We were closer in age, had the same mother and father, and had experienced much of the same negative experiences with our older siblings. It was a good thing he came. We got into a very heated argument with Derek, who proceeded to put his finger in my face, and when I went to remove his finger, he attempted to slap me. The next thing I know, a full brawl had broken out. Me and Mark against Derek and Michael. I know it sounds crazy and even embarrassing that we would be fighting at a funeral home, but when I think about it and how they have been all of my life, it was not that strange. In fact, it had been a long time coming, and it was much overdue. We would spend the next year and a half dealing with the court which brought legal charges against both of them. Although they did not suffer any major consequences from the judicial system, they were banned from attending my sister's memorial, and given a strong warning to never bother me again. It was the final encounter I would ever have to experience with them, and I was relieved and glad. Nevertheless, the year did not end as well as it had started. I had attended school for one semester, and I was doing well in my two classes; however, like clockwork, my depressive symptoms returned. I am not sure if it was the winter blues, my sister's death, the fight with my older siblings, or a combination of all three, but here I was struggling again. I had been planning a women's summit, something the Lord had placed upon my heart to do in my home city, but I canceled it due to my sister's death and all of the chaos surrounding it.

When the second semester of my first year started in January of 2018, I was very low. It was a tremendous struggle for me to go to class. I felt like I was in a fog for a few months. But then once again, things became better, and I went on with my life. Things got even better that spring. I had returned to the gym and had started exercising and losing weight again due to the interest two men had expressed toward me. That was something I had not experienced for some time. It felt good to be desired. The fall of 2018 was a peak period for me. I was doing well at work and in school. I was losing weight and beginning to feel better about myself again. I was doing all of the things I desired and that I thought would keep me happy and well. And yet, when the winter came, I once again found myself experiencing major depressive symptoms. It became so bad I decided to step away from work and school the spring semester of 2019. I was successful with taking time off from work, but I allowed my professor to talk me out of taking time off from school. I had her the previous semester, and she thought very highly of me. She appreciated my writing ability as well as my participation in class. She encouraged me to continue in the program and said she would give me the support I needed to thrive throughout the semester. She would allow me to miss class when I needed to and to submit work after the deadline when necessary. I had her for both of my classes, so that was a blessing. I took a leave of absence from teaching, but I continued with school where I attended classes and also participated in a practicum that literally took the life out of me. Unlike education, where the practicum experience is at the end of the program, the practicum for the social work program would coincide with taking classes. It was difficult to manage, and I was extremely disappointed in my assignments. The first semester mainly consisted of me writing out these twenty-page assessments I had done with clients at the facility in which I served. Other than that, I had no hands on experience. The second semester, my assignment was changed, and it was even worse. The program I was assigned to was a great program, but my role in the program was extremely insignificant. I merely took attendance set-up refreshments and entered data from surveys. It was something a teenager could have done, and it was not giving me any real practice in the mental health field, none that I desired. When I entered the MSSW program, I stressed the fact that I worked full-time and my concern that my practicum experiences would not be as fulfilling due to my schedule and my inability to serve during the daytime. I was assured that this program was suitable for working adults like me, but I found this to not be truthful at all. After my second year, I decided to take some time off. I was still dealing with depressive symptoms. I had run out of money so I had to return to work, and I knew I could not do both work and school at this time. I remember my brother, his wife at the time, and in-laws trying to encourage me to keep going. I had made it to my third and final year, but they had no idea what I was experiencing or how I felt.

Everyone experiences depression differently. Most people think depression is simply being sad and that it is something you can snap yourself out of. That may be others' experience, but it was not mine. The reason I had gone so many years not knowing it was depression was because of the way it surfaced for me. There are several major symptoms I experience, which include severe fatigue, disorganization, brain fogginess, feelings of being overwhelmed, hopelessness, and sometimes suicide ideation. I was experiencing all of these in 2019, but not to the degree that I had when I found myself in that hotel room. Although, I was not able to do much of anything. I crawled out of the bed to attend my classes, which were still held in the evening, and to attend my practicum, and that was it. I was so glad when the semester was over. For whatever reason, for many years, I had always struggled with returning to work in the fall. But like clockwork, once the school year resumed that fall, I was fine. It is like once I get back into the swing of things and establish a routine, I begin to feel better. Sadly, that only last a few months before the winter blues return, which I later learned was Seasonal Affective Disorder. I also had to learn that it does not just occur during the winter months, but it can occur during the summer months also, which I had also experienced. But I went back to work because I had to be able to take care of myself. The school year of 2019-2020 was the hardest school year for me, and this was well before the Covid-19 Pandemic hit. I felt so out of the loop, unprepared, and unable to keep up with my peers. Any new information that they threw at us, whether it was a new program or new technology, I felt extremely overwhelmed. I cried a lot. I would even have panic attacks. One day, I had one at work. I had a few challenging classes that semester, and I felt like I had lost control. One day, right before class, I had begun to feel very anxious. The lesson activity I had prepared would only last for about half of the class, and I knew because of that I would lose even more control of the class. I had begun to feel nervous about the possibility of me having an unscheduled observation by one of my administrators and me being unprepared and receiving a poor evaluation. When the bell rang, I remember walking to my door to greet the students. I remember a student walking up to me and her asking me what was wrong. I did not realize it, but tears had begun to pour down my face. I put both hands over my mouth. I felt as though I was going to scream. I walked two doors down to one of my neighbors with my hands covering my mouth and tears still streaming down my face. I remember my colleague asking me what was wrong, but I could not speak. She called an administrator who eventually called the school nurse who confirmed I was more than likely having a panic attack. I was so embarrassed. I finally got myself together but was encouraged to go home for the remainder of the day to rest, and so I did. That would not be the last time I experienced that feeling of anxiety and panic at work. There were several days I would get to work and maybe teach for a class period or two before calling the secretary and telling her I needed someone to cover my classroom so I could leave. I remember leaving work many days and stopping by the store to purchase some sort of sleep aid so I could just take something and go to sleep. I could not even deal with what was happening to me. This may sound crazy, but when Covid-19 hit, I was very relieved. I was not completely aware of what it was and the impact it would have. All I knew was that school was going to be shut down for, what they believed at this time, three whole weeks. I had convinced myself I just needed rest and that once I felt rested, I would feel my second wind and would be able to finish out the year strong. I would take a week to rest, and then use the other two weeks to do some lesson planning, something I had not been able to do for a long time. I was literally just going day to day. I was faking my way through, hoping I would not be found out. Only thing is, the virus was more than we realized. School would not reopen, and I wouldn't leave my bed. It was the darkest time of my life. Even as I write this, I am still not ready to share about it. So, I will leave this here, until I am ready to share more.

CHAPTER 3

Let Me Back Up

Now that I know more about depression, anxiety, and other areas of mental health, I would say I have always had issues I just did not have a name for them. Even in my childhood, I remember things I experienced, both circumstantially and emotionally. I honestly do not know where to begin to explain my family background. I will do my best to share in the shortest amount of time possible. My mother had me later in life. She was forty-one years old. My father, however, was twenty-nine years old. They met when they both worked together at the Veteran's Hospital in Louisville, Kentucky. I have heard so many different stories about their meeting. I can only share what I have heard and what I believe to be true. From what I understand, my mother was married when she met my father. She entered a relationship with my father and after becoming pregnant with my brother Mark, she left her husband. It was shared with me that her marriage was very abusive both physically and verbally. Her husband was what you would call a true "hell raiser". He would become upset about anything. His children, my older siblings, and my mother feared and even hated him to a certain degree. Still, she remained with him for almost twenty years. Maybe it was because of the time period in which she lived. They married because she was pregnant. I am sure she also loved him. But, during those times, men were the breadwinners and sole providers. My mother is no longer living, so I do not have her to verify what I am sharing here; so, I am doing my best. When she found out she was pregnant and had decided to enter a full relationship with my father, she left her husband. In addition to being pregnant, she also had four older children-three boys and a girl. I believe her divorce became final sometime after having my brother Mark and shortly before I was born. My parents were in a relationship and lived together until I was about five years old. I have very little memory of him living with us, but I do remember him being there and him leaving. I remember being extremely sad when he left. My father was my caretaker. He was declared medically disabled the year I was born. So, he stayed home and took care of me while my mother worked. My father wanted to marry my mother, but they never did because of his mental illness. In fact, that was the reason for their relationship ending. My father was diagnosed with what would later be known as Bipolar I Disorder. He had periods of extreme depression and random episodes of mania. I have heard stories of him destroying things in our home, taking money, and flying to a different state on a whim. He had been previously married and had a son a little less than two years before Mark was born. As I grew older, I learned to not fault my mother for not remaining with my father. In her eyes, she was protecting my brother Mark and me. They maintained a good friendship, and my father was allowed and encouraged to maintain a relationship with Mark and me. He was always welcome in our home, during holidays and as he pleased. We even still did some family things together, such as go to the movies. I was very much a daddy's girl. I did not understand his illness until much later and could not understand why I could not live with my father. From my perspective, he lived much better than me. He and my grandmother shared an apartment, along with a few of my cousins from time to time. The times I would spend at my grandmother and father's home were the best. Their home was clean. The children who lived there had chores, and I would assist when I was there. I liked it because it provided structure, something I have learned in my experience as an educator for twenty plus years that all children truly desire. There was always something to eat in their refrigerator, and my grandmother cooked supper every day. My father did fun things with us, such as taking us to Chuck E Cheese, to putt putt golf, and swimming. I lived for the time I would be with my father. The only thing is I would be a little sad and felt a little guilty being there. I would remember my mother being home, and I would feel so sorry for her. Three of my older siblings Michael, Michelle (Shellie), and Derek lived there; even though they were old enough to live on their own.

Our home was depressing and chaotic. It was hardly ever clean, unless I cleaned it. My mother hardly cooked meals. My brother Mark and I lived off hotdogs, bologna, and French fries made from real potatoes. My siblings were oftentimes in trouble with the law and/or fighting one another. It seemed like every time we turned around, someone was in jail. They had taken much after their father's side of the family which wreaked with alcoholism, drug addiction, and criminal behavior. Derek was the most troubled child my mother had. He is thirteen years older than me. He used to be my favorite sibling. I loved him tremendously. When my mother and father separated, he became the father or male role. He would babysit my brother Mark and me while my mother worked. There was always something going on with Derek, and him getting into trouble started very early, before teenage years even. He stole from the neighbors and even stole from our family. I remember one time him stealing our VCR while we were still at home. On three different occasions, he was stabbed in the streets. I am not completely sure what brought on the fights he had with other people, but he never seemed to win any of them. He was stabbed in his arm with a pitchfork, in his hand with a bottle that was intended for his head, and in his chest by a guy who was supposedly his best friend. He almost died that time. In fact, they pronounced him dead and told my mother that he was. Miraculously, he recovered from all three incidents, but that did not stop him from living a life of criminal activity. He was a thief and not very good at it. My mother would spend all her money on bailing him out of jail. She even put up our house a few times as bond. She eventually lost her house because of that. I remember being and doing without so many things as a child because of Derek. As I mentioned, at one point, he was my favorite. He was a senior when I was in kindergarten. Every day when he ran to catch the bus to school, I would literally stand in the door and cry because I could not understand why he had to leave me. Never in a million years would I have imagined the pain he would cause my family and me. At some point, I learned to not care for him as much as I did. I think I did that to protect myself. I felt that one day he would get hurt and would not live through it, and I tried to prepare my heart to live without him. Because my mother always ran to his aid, I felt that he was her favorite. She would not let him feel the sting of his poor actions, not even a little bit. Even as a child, I would think that maybe if she did not rescue him as quickly just one time that he would straighten up.

I had a lot of shame as a child. I was embarrassed by my family and by our home. Friends were never allowed to come over because there was not any room for them. For years, I shared a room and bed with my sister who was eighteen years older than me. There were times when she would disappear, and we did not know where she was. I am sure my mother was saddened and worried, but those were happy times for me because it would mean I would have my own bedroom to myself. My bedroom was my safe space. I had hidden there when fights broke out between my siblings. I would just spend a lot of time in there because it meant being away from everyone else. My bedroom was not the nicest. I never had new bedroom furniture or anything. But I kept it clean, and I kept in there the things I felt I needed. At one time, I had a small black and white TV my father had bought me. Somehow, it came up missing. I believe Derek stole and sold it as he did anything worth any value in our home. I remember being sad and alone a lot of times. Mark was two and half years older than me, and he was a boy; so, he was allowed to do certain things before me and things I just simply was not allowed to do because I was a girl. My mother had little control over him after a certain age. I cried a lot and dreamt of living a better life with my dad. He would come and visit and take my mind off of what was going on in my home, but that was only temporarily.

I knew about God. My mother took us to church where I attended Sunday school. I even attended Vacation Bible School with my friends at our neighborhood church. In high school, I joined a youth group that was facilitated by a local church. My daddy would even talk to me about saying my prayers and told me he prayed for me every night. Yet, my heart was repeatedly broken. I could not understand why God would allow me to be born into such a family. Why couldn't I live a normal life like my friends appeared to live? Why did I have to go hungry? Why did I have to go without the things I wanted and even sometimes the essentials because my mother was too busy trying to rescue a son that had no intentions of being saved? Even my sister was a problem. All three of my older siblings that lived in the home drank alcohol and used drugs. And none of them worked consistently. Michael worked a part-time job at a Kroger's for a while. Eventually, he went on to work at a hotel. He did not receive his high school diploma or his G.E.D., so I am sure there were not many higher paying jobs he could do. My sister once worked for a barbeque restaurant and did very well there for a while, enough to buy herself a car. I am not sure why none of them had the desire or motivation to move out on their own. My mother did not push them either. It was like they had some kind of hold over her that she could not release them nor hold them to any level of accountability. Many years later, I would ask my mother why she never made them stand up, Shellie especially. I remember watching her as tears filled her eyes, and although she did admit there was some kind of hold my sister had over her, she would never tell me what it was. Maybe she felt guilty for all of the years she subjected them to living with their father. I said he was a hell raiser. He would fight my mother and discipline my brothers and sister. It would be considered abuse today. My mother and siblings always talked about their old home, 36th Street. They always talked about how nice it was, how they had nice things, and how they kept it clean or else. I wonder if that is why my home was never kept clean. Maybe my mother was tired of doing so after what she endured with her husband. Maybe it was because there was no one there to keep things in check, even if it was done violently. Nevertheless, I was miserable as a child.

On two different occasions, I took a bunch of pills. I am not sure if I was trying to commit suicide or not. I never told anyone about it. I was in the seventh grade both times I did it. The first time, my sister was suspicious. I slept in every class period at school, and when I came home, I immediately went to bed. I remember my sister waking me up and looking me over. She asked what was wrong with me. I told her we had dissected a worm or a frog (I can't remember which one) and that it had made me sick to my stomach. I am not sure if she believed me or not, but she let me be. I slept it off and continued as if nothing had happened. I have oftentimes wondered what would have happened had I not gone to school that day. Like, what if I had taken the pills on a Friday night and the next day was Saturday. Would I have just been left to sleep and never waken up? Would I have died? Although I can be thankful for that now, there was a time where I was actually disappointed that was not the case. I never really had the boldness to end my own life, but I did not want to live either. I believed in heaven and would have rather been there than living the life I was living. It was not until I got to high school that things became better, mainly because I was not at home as much.

My oldest nephew, Adrian, came to live with us when I was twelve years old. Ever since he had been born and even more so now, I had to babysit him when my mother worked. This was really burdensome during the summertime when I wanted to just be free and hang with my friends. Instead, I was busy taking care of him. I was only six years older than him, but I still had to take care of him not his father, Michael, and not Mark who was older than me, but me. I was the girl, and my sister was absent at this time. Every day, I would wake up, get us both dressed, and go to the recreation center, which was the elementary school's gymnasium. I would talk to my friends while he played and ate free lunch. When we got home, I would be hungry by then, so I would fry us some potatoes or whatever else I could find in the refrigerator. There was not much. I had volunteered with my mother a few summers and realized that partly why my mother was not as concerned about what we ate at home was because she ate while at work. After a few years, I got tired of taking care of my nephew. I had been so excited when we learned about him and becoming an aunt. My excitement quickly faded because he was made to be my responsibility, and although I loved him very much, I did not think that was fair. The end of my freshman year, I decided to do something about it. I figured I was only required to babysit because I was available and that if I became unavailable, I would not have to do so. I met a good friend name Kenya Roberts, who I say to this day changed the trajectory of my life. She convinced me and some of our other friends to try out for the dance team and for color guard with the marching band. We all made color guard, but I was the only one to make the dance team. That summer, I got out of babysitting because of the practices I had. I was relieved. Once the school year began, I became even more unavailable at home, I began participating in school clubs and the youth chapter of the local NAACP. My junior year, I got a part-time job. Between my practices and working, I was hardly ever home, but when I was, I still hated it. By this time, my older siblings had moved out, but someone was always moving back home. On one occasion, my sister even moved her boyfriend home with her. Of course, they took over my bedroom, and once again, I had to share a bed with my mother. When I was younger, I would spend a lot of time at my friend Sherry's home. I loved being there. Their house was clean, they had a mother and a father in the home, there was always something good to eat, and it was always fun without any negative drama. I learned a lot from that family. I learned about my period and biology. They were the family I wished I had. I remember one night them staying up to explain to me that growing up does not mean you have to get stabbed. That is what I truly believed because of my experience with my older brother. I lived in fear with that for a while. This family, along with sports, school and community clubs, and a few good friends were a huge distraction and comfort for me. They gave me the relief and the hope I needed that one day I would be able to leave my family and my home behind.

I had wanted to be a school teacher for as long as I could remember. I loved school, and when I was not at school, I was making all the neighborhood friends play school with me. I would always be the teacher. Once I figured out, I had to go to college in order to become a teacher that became my sole focus. It would be my way to finally escape the hell I lived in at home. The sad part is that some people had an idea of the dysfunction I grew up in, but many had no clue whatsoever. Things became much better when I got a boyfriend the end of my junior year. I practically lived at my boyfriend Trico's home. He would come and get me, and once I got a car, I would drive there every opportunity I had. His home was what I desired. It was clean, there was always food, and he and his sister had chores, which I would help with when it was his turn. Looking back on that, it probably was not wise to allow two teenagers to spend as much time together as we did in his bedroom, but it was my safe haven. Even Trico understood the sadness I lived with at home. I remember him coming over one time and me refusing to allow him into my house. He thought I was hiding someone; he did not realize I was hiding something. My house was a mess, and I was embarrassed. I think by this time, I had grown tired of trying to keep it clean. Sadly, and I have not said this until now, my mother was the one who kept it filthy. I remember one summer literally cleaning the majority of the house daily, and then her coming home and messing it back up every single day. I am not saying I did not have any good childhood memories at home. Nor am I saying my mother did not love me. I guess she did the best she could. I am not sure. I know I was loved. Maybe she was dealing with my older siblings so much she just did not have the time nor strength to be concerned about me or Mark. I think it was different for me though because I was a girl. I saw the relationship some of my friends had with their mothers. I desperately wanted that, but I knew I would never have it because she just did not have enough to give to all of us. I was angry about it for much of my childhood. It was not until I graduated from college that I was able to confront her about that. Why were Mark and I denied clothes and other nice things because she had to do for grown children? Why would she sacrifice the bad children for the good children? I remember one time when I was home on a break from college, my brother Derek's girlfriend at the time telling my mother that he had gotten the money she sent to him. He was in jail at the time; when was he not? This made me extremely angry and hurt because I remember asking her for money that summer for food and her telling me she did not have any. I had attended summer school. During the academic year when you lived in the dorms, room and board included meals, but this was not the case during the summer months. I did not know this initially. So, I had to buy and cook my own groceries. As I am writing this, I realize this is more than likely when my weight issues began because of the food choices I had to make. I remember eating rice and other filling food during that time. And to come home and hear that she sent fifty dollars to my brother who was in jail for something he had done and not for the first or final time was extremely disheartening. Here I was in college trying to make something of myself and make her proud, but she was still giving her all, including her money, to those who did nothing to appreciate it. The good thing about it was that as sad and as angry as I was and had the right to be, this made me go even harder. I had something to prove. I had to prove I could make it, even without her full support, and that I would grow up to be nothing like her or my older siblings.

During college, I became more serious about my faith in Jesus Christ. I had become a member of a gospel choir called Voices of Triumph and had started attending Bible studies and church on my own. I was learning more about God and had truly begun to see how he had been keeping me all of these years. I knew before Marvin Sapp wrote the song that I never would have made it without Him and that because of Him, I truly was stronger, wiser, and better. I was everything my siblings were not nor could ever be. In part, I felt like it was a result of my hard work and ambition, but I began to learn more and more about the grace and mercy of God and that without Him, my efforts would not have mattered. On the day I left home to go to college, I made a vow to myself that I would never come back to live in that house again and celebrated that I was finally free. So, when I graduated from college, I knew where I would go, anywhere but back home. I had obtained a grant which I had committed to remaining in Indiana to teach for three years, so I sought out a place to live that was in Indiana but further away from Jeffersonville. I did not really care for Indianapolis. It was a little too big and confusing for me. I had a sorority sister who went to Fort Wayne and a few friends who were from there, so I decided to give it a shot. I interviewed with two school districts and was hired by the second one. This was another decision and opportunity that changed the trajectory of my life. I was somewhat afraid to leave the comforts of the community I had created in college, but I knew I had to go out into the real world. I made a decision that in addition to teaching, I would use this as an opportunity to continue my spiritual growth, and that I did. About a year after college, I heard and accepted the calling of God to preach the Gospel of Jesus Christ. However, I felt that something was holding me back. The anger and resentment I had toward my mother. I had tried to address some of it while I was in college. I remember meeting with a campus counselor on one occasion, and I remember meeting with the minister and leader of the gospel choir as well. This time, I would go to my pastor. Through much counsel and prayer, I decided to confront my mother about the thoughts and feelings I had toward her. I wanted to empty my heart of the negativity so I could go forth and be all I believed God was calling me to be. I was too afraid to have the conversation over the telephone or face-to-face, so I wrote a twenty plus page letter and fearfully waited until she received and read it. Those were the longest days ever. When she finally received it and called me, I was too afraid to answer her call, so I let it go to my answering machine. She was extremely upset and very defensive. We did not talk about it at that time because I had done exactly what I did not want to do. I had hurt my mother. As hurt as I was, I never wanted to hurt her. But it was necessary. I had to tell her my truth. I told her about how she repeatedly chose my older siblings over me. I told her about how I went without so much of what I needed, including her, because she was too busy trying to fix them. I even pointed out the time she sent my brother fifty dollars when he was in jail and how it took her three weeks to send my twenty-six dollars in my sister's food stamps. Everything I shared was truthful, and I tried to do it respectfully. I even had my pastor read the letter to make sure it was not intentionally hurtful. I also assigned him with the task of putting it in the mail for fear I would not be able to do it. As time went on, I realized the apology and acknowledgement I wanted from my mother would never come. The next time I saw her, I knew she would act as though nothing had happened and that I would go along with it. However, there was an Evangelist who came to our church one time, and during the message, I felt strongly led to forgive my mother. If I was going to preach the Gospel, I could not preach one thing and live another. I could not tell others to forgive when I had not forgiven my mother. I picked up the telephone and called my mother. When she answered, I told her that although she may never ask for it, that I forgave her for hurting me. What a relief that was. She eventually wrote a letter to me where in her own way, she acknowledged my pain and an explanation regarding the decisions she made during my upbringing. Primarily, she stated that my older siblings were her weaker children and that I was her strong child. She said she needed to be there more for them because they needed her and that she knew I would be okay. I have a good friend, Sheryl, who has reiterated to me numerous times how mothers know their children and they know what each of them needs. Although I did not agree with that, I accepted it, and I forgave her. I am not sure if I truly let it go then, as I would still struggle with the attention and devotion my mother gave to my older siblings over me, but I was stronger now. There was always an imaginary line that separated me from them. For whatever reason, they were resentful towards Mark and me. We knew it, and we felt it. I guess we both did the best we could to survive that and thrive in spite of it. The number of adverse childhood experiences I had most definitely impacted my mental health. Both fortunately and unfortunately, I was able to suppress those effects for a while, until I no longer could.

CHAPTER 4
I Put A Name To It

It was in 2009 that I was finally able to put a name to what it was that I had been experiencing. At this point, I had been thriving as an adult. I was a teacher. I was serving in ministry. I had my own condo. I was very well-established. Sometime between 2003 and 2006, I remember having these episodes where I would get extremely fatigued. Initially and for a long while, I thought it was burnout. That was a buzz word at the time, and I certainly fit the description. I was working full-time, and even though I was not getting paid for it, I was serving full-time in ministry as well. I had ministerial responsibilities at my church, and I also was the visionary and leader for a women's ministry which I founded. I believe around this time that I was also pursuing my first master's degree. I would literally leave work and then go serve in some ministry capacity, whether that was attending and participating in a worship service, attending, and potentially leading a meeting, or hosting a Bible study or event. Anyone who knows about the profession of teaching also understands that the job does not end when you leave the building. I had work to grade, lessons to plan, and assignments and assessments to create. Because I was also a student, I had books to read, notes to study, and papers and projects to complete. So, experiencing burn out was not a strange assumption to have. When I would experience these episodes of feeling fatigue and overwhelmed, I would share with my dear friend and sister, Michele. She would typically pray with me, and eventually it would lift, and I would feel better. Only, the episodes started happening more often. I was not sure what to do. I thought that perhaps I needed to take some things off of my plate, which was wise to do. I remember at the start of one year making a list of all of the things I did in ministry. I then separated the list into two columns. In the first column, I listed the things I believed I was gifted and called to do. In the second column, I listed the things I did either out of obligation or enjoyment. When I first got serious about ministry, I was not quite sure what my gifts were or where to serve in ministry, and so I did a little bit of everything. Soon, I became known for serving in these areas and for many, I was almost expected to continue to do these things. There are not many capacities in which I have not served in the local church: youth ministry coordinator, radio ministry leader, helps ministry, choir, praise team, finance office, secretarial staff, women's ministry, singles ministry, Christian education, church announcements I did a lot. When I finished my list, I determined that I was mostly gifted and called in the area of teaching, administration, and leadership. So, I gave up a lot of things; even something that I truly enjoyed, singing in the choir and on the praise team. I just did not have the time or the energy to attend all the meetings and rehearsals that were required. I thought that narrowing down my responsibilities would remedy the fatigue episodes I was experiencing, but essentially, it did not.

At some point, I decided to talk to my primary care physician about what I was experiencing. I remember him suggesting that I was possibly experiencing symptoms of depression and recommending that I begin taking an antidepressant. I was completely shocked and did not agree with him at all. I was not depressed. I was not sad about anything or having crying spells. I knew a little bit about depression from my father's experience, and I was nothing like that. I was a fully functioning adult. I had a career and was serving God to the best of my ability. I had aspirations to work and be paid to do ministry full-time. Surely God was with me and pleased with me, and I was not depressed because of it. I am not sure if it was my doctor's recommendation or how it came about, but before taking medication, I agreed to see a therapist. My friend Michele recommended one to me. Her name was Cathy. When I first began therapy, I do not believe that behavioral health was covered by my insurance. So, she allowed payment on a sliding scale. I paid $50 per visit. I believe that my initial commitment was to see her every other week. She was a great help to me. Through her, I realized that there was a lot from my childhood and even in my young adulthood that I had not confronted. I had simply suppressed everything so that I could continue moving forward, and I guess it was slowly but surely beginning to seep out. We attacked things that I experienced in my childhood. For the first time, I was given permission to be angry and to address the traumatic experiences I had as a child. I shared with her about how I hated my siblings and how they made growing up extremely miserable. I shared with her about how angry I was that my father had succumbed to his mental illness after losing his mother, my grandmother, and how I felt like I did not have anyone else to love and look out for me the way that he did. I told her about the Pastor who was supposed to be that father figure for me, how I had seen him as a teacher and a protector, and how I was angry because of the sexual relationship that he initiated with me but how I was left carrying the weight of it. I was viewed to be this seductive young woman who took advantage of him, and that was not the case at all. I was a young woman, and he was eighteen years my senior. I had opened up to him about some resentment that I carried toward my family. He was very aware of that, and he used my vulnerability to satisfy his own lustful desires. I was made to feel that I could not tell anyone of leadership or authority because they loved him and would protect him at all costs. I left the church, and he just went on as if nothing had happened. My world was destroyed. I could not even tell my mother. She had suspected something before anything ever began. I remember being extremely angry about her suspicions as well as others. He was my Pastor, and he would never do that. Looking back at it now, it was very much predatory. He studied me, and he lured me right where he wanted. He elevated me in various areas of ministry which he knew I aspired to. I became the radio ministry coordinator, and I wrote for the broadcasts that he recorded. We worked together a lot recording the broadcasts. One summer, he even paid me to assist in the church's office with record keeping and other things. He had gone through a divorce, so he was single, and he had full custody of his two children. Like others in the church, I wanted to lighten the load. I started doing things for him, such as taking him lunch, never realizing that my intentions were being perceived incorrectly. He would invite me to his home, and I would spend time with him there as well outside of church. Eventually, our relationship became romantic. This went on for a while before I left the church and even long after that. It took me a long time to realize that I had been taken advantage of and that our relationship was completely inappropriate, but that I was not the seducer, I was the seduced. Cathy and I talked about a lot of things. It felt good to finally confront things I had buried inside of me for such a long time. I began to feel better. But soon, the same feelings of fatigue and feeling overwhelmed would return. Cathy began teaching me about depression, the different areas of the brain in which it affects, and how different medications treat it. It took a while for me to commit to taking medication. I had briefly mentioned it to my mother, and she told me that I did not need medicine. Knowing my mother's thoughts as well as the thoughts of others in the church who had been very vocal against medication for mental illness, I fought long and hard not to take anything.

By 2008, my desire to serve full-time in ministry had grown even more. I had a different Pastor at this time. I had learned a different method of teaching and really desired to become an even greater teacher of the Word of God. I believed that God was calling me to the Pastorate, and I wanted to attend a seminary to obtain a Master of Divinity so that I could have a true understanding of the Word. I began doing some research to see what schools were out there and where my study could take me. At this time, I was desiring to leave Fort Wayne. I loved the work I was doing in ministry, but I no longer wanted to be a classroom teacher. It was never my intention to remain in Fort Wayne, Indiana, for as long as I had. In fact, Fort Wayne did not even become an option until I was preparing to graduate from Ball State University. I needed a job, but I had no idea where to go. I had received a grant for minority teachers, and part of the agreement was that I would teach in the state of Indiana for three years. Although I was not quite sure where to go, I knew where I did not want to go. I did not want to return home to Jeffersonville. I also did not want to move to Indianapolis. It was too big and intimidating for me. I had a possible opportunity to teach at the school where I had done my student teaching in Anderson, but I felt I would be too close to Ball State. Some things had happened at the end of my senior year, and I wanted to put some distance between me and some of the people there. I also remember feeling very afraid to leave college. It had become my home and safety net for the past four years. I felt that if I would have taken the job in Anderson that I would have been in Muncie all of time and that I would have had an even harder time cutting ties in order for me to grow into an independent adult. One of my sorority sisters had taken a job in Fort Wayne. I knew a few people from there. One of my roommates was from there. So, I gave it a try, and I got the job. The plan was to teach there for three years and then to move elsewhere, but I ended up staying. I bought my first condo after my fourth year, and I was adopted by a family that took me in as their own. And so, Fort Wayne became home for me. When I would go home to visit my family, I could not wait to return home to Fort Wayne, away from all of the dysfunction within my family and the reminders of all that I had endured as a child. But by this time, I felt I had outgrown Fort Wayne, and I was ready to leave. Memphis, Tennessee, had been an area I had considered when searching for my first teaching job. It was still close to my hometown, about five and a half hours away. I went to a job interview and was offered a job, but I turned it down.

At the start of 2009, I went on a fast as I pondered if this was what God would have me to do. At the end of the fast, I felt that God was in agreement, and so I decided to pursue this opportunity. I shared with my Pastor, I put my condo up for sale, I resigned from my job, and I made preparations to move. It was an exciting time, and yet, this is when my world began to crumble the first time. I was experiencing the fatigue a lot more frequently, and the episodes were lasting much longer. I also began to experience anxiety at this time because I realized that I was around the same age as my father when depression overtook his life. I was afraid. I did not know what was going on with me, and I could not tell anyone. And the one person I felt I could tell, Michele, was preparing to leave Fort Wayne to take another job. She had also met her now husband, and so although we were still close in spirit and I knew that she loved me deeply as her friend and sister, her focus was elsewhere. I felt extremely alone. I was ashamed. How was I to be this great and strong minister who had ministered to others about the power of God, and yet here I was struggling. What would others say if they knew? What would they think of me? What does this mean? Does this mean that my faith is weak? Am I being punished for the ongoing sexual relationship I had with the Pastor? Was this hereditary and something that I would now deal with for the remainder of my life? Was I being oppressed by demonic spirits? I had consulted one other person about these episodes before, Prophet Daniel Byrd, my spiritual father, but by this time, he had lost his wife and was struggling to live through that. I did not want to burden him even more, and I was not sure if he could handle it. And so, I remained silent. I began to isolate myself away from everyone. I believe that others had begun to see the change in me, but they too did not know what to think, say, or do. With the group of sister friends that I had in my women's ministry, I did not feel I could go to any of them because of the way in which they esteemed me. I did not want to let any of them down. I felt as though people saw what was going on with me but that they became afraid of me, and so they stayed away from me as well. And then, I am sure that some were hurt by the fact that I was leaving Fort Wayne, thus walking away from them and the ministry we had built together, even if it was to do an even greater work for the Lord. My condo became extremely messy. The only time I would somewhat clean is if I was having a showing to sell my condo, and that was not going very well. By this time, I knew that I was depressed, but I could not figure out why. I was not sure if it was because things were not going according to my plan, which was to sell my condo and live off the profit for at least the first year of school, or if it was something I would have experienced no matter what. That became a huge burden that I would endure for many years when I would have episodes trying to figure out the cause. My condo was not selling, and I had resigned from my job. I did not know what I was going to do if the condo did not sell. Even more worrisome was having to find another job and the embarrassment I would face by saying that I heard from God yet things were not working out. What would that say about me then? Had I truly heard from God, or was this just something I wanted and set out to do on my own? Was I out of God's will? In addition to not being able to keep my home clean, I was also falling behind on paying my bills. I had gone months without paying bills. I had the money. I just did not have the energy to sit down and write out the checks. This was before online banking.

I am not sure how honest I was being with my therapist about what was going on with me. Because it was summertime, I was not working. And so, I did not really have a reason to get out of bed to do anything or go anywhere. I had stepped away from my church responsibilities as well as the ministry that I led outside of the church. I literally stayed in bed and watched television and slept. I did not see anyone for weeks at a time. At one time, the only interaction I had was with Michele's now husband, Alvin. I paid him to paint various rooms in my condo. I am not sure what his thoughts were when he would come and find me in the bed. By this time, I had let my cable go to save money, and so I would simply watch VHS tapes and DVDs. At one point, I did finally reach out to my mother and asked her to come, but once again, I was disappointed. I am not sure why she could never really come when I felt that I needed her. And it was rare that I would actually express to her that I did. Maybe it was because of the fear she had of being away from my older siblings and what would possibly happen while she was away. Maybe it was the burden of having to be there to support them. Maybe it was because she rarely had any extra money to make the trip because of her taking care of them. I just know that when I needed her, she was not there for me, and I was devastated. That, I would say, was my first rock bottom. I had been slacking on going to therapy, as it was becoming a major expense. Somehow, I went to see Cathy. I believe she started allowing me to come without paying the previous bill. We talked again about taking medication, and this time, I was willing. I had to do something. I was not ready to share it with other people yet, but I was tired of feeling the way I felt and living the way I was living. I was willing to do whatever I could to feel like my normal self again. I was tired of suffering, tired of being alone, tired of being afraid. I needed help, and if medicine was going to help me, I could no longer refuse. I would be treated for Major Depressive Disorder.

I began taking the medication and going to therapy. I was getting a lot out of therapy and dealing with a lot of my trauma, particularly from my childhood and from the inappropriate relationship I shared with the Pastor. My condo still had not sold, and I was not sure about my plans working out for me to still leave to attend seminary, but I seemed to begin feeling a lot better. I felt so much better that I did what many people make the mistake of doing I stopped taking my medication abruptly. I have since learned that is a huge no, no, and the side effects from it. As a result, I experienced what would be my first hypomanic episode. Hypomania is a form of mania but not to the same degree. I had witnessed mania before with my father; so, I never for once thought my behavior was abnormal. Suddenly, I had more energy than I had experienced in a long time. My mother did finally come to visit me, and by having her support, I was able to commit to pursuing a part-time adjunct position as an instructor at a local college. This would allow me to begin earning income again, and precisely the amount I needed to cover my debt. My only concern during this time was not having health insurance. Yet, I was hopeful I could at least maintain until my home sold. By this time, the school year had begun, and so it was too late for me to try to return to my old job. Besides, I was certain that someone had already taken the position; it had been months since I had resigned. I was still somewhat ashamed that my plan had not worked, and so I continued to isolate from my friends. I am not sure what their thoughts were of me. At this time, there were only two people who even slightly knew what was going on with me, my friends Terri and Natasha. They had both been active members in the women's ministry I had founded and oversaw for several years. When I had gotten extremely depressed and things were really bad, my therapist had encouraged me to solicit their support. I eventually called on them, mainly to help me write the checks to pay my bills and to clean my condo. It was hard bringing them into my darkness, but when asked, neither hesitated to help me. Terri and I were more familiar with one another, but Tasha and I had started to become closer. She was going to take over the women's ministry that I was leaving behind as the new leader, and I trusted that it was in great hands. Natasha and I started spending more time together, and I believe she was able to see more of what I was dealing with more than anyone else. By this time, I felt abandoned. I felt that no one really saw what I was going through and those that did thought that I was struggling simply because my condo had not sold, and my plans had not worked out. But that was not it. I realized years later that even if my condo had sold that I would have still been depressed. In fact, things might have turned out worse because I would have probably still tried to continue with my plan even though I no longer had the stamina to fulfill it. During this hypomanic phrase, I made a horrible decision to enter a relationship that had I been well, I would have never even considered. He was the brother of one of my very good friends, Carmen. I had become a part of their family, and so we had been around one another for several years. The enemy is crafty. He waited until my thinking was distorted, my guard was down, and I was extremely vulnerable to send this relationship. His name was Rodney. In my right mind, I would have never even looked at Rodney. The primary reason was because we were like family, but also, Rodney was not even on my level. Rodney was about five years older than me but had very little going for himself. It was well-known that he was a womanizer. He was never faithful in his past relationships. He had five children by five different women, three of which were around the same age. He had been dishonorably discharged from the military due to his misbehavior, and now, he was back home living in between his parents and different women. One day, he sent me a text telling me that he wanted to take me on a date before I left. It was something he said he had always wanted to do. I am not sure why t, but I did not see the harm in this. I was still planning to leave Fort Wayne to attend seminary once my condo sold, and I was completely unaware of Rodney's true intentions. I allowed him to visit me once when my mother had come to visit. He brought my godson and his brother with him. I did not think anything of it, but my mother saw what was going on; mothers always know. I still saw Rodney like a family member and would have never thought that he had other intentions. Even though he was not much of a good catch, he was cool and very fun to be around. Anytime he was ever around, we were bound to have a lot of laughs. He was always the life of the party. I agreed to allow him to take me on a date to dinner and a movie, but before that, for some reason, I allowed him to come spend the night. I knew that nothing would happen because for one, I was on my menstrual cycle. After allowing him to spend the night, things moved rather quickly between us. We became sexually involved, and before I knew it, for the first time in over a decade, I had a boyfriend. I turned into a woman that

I had always despised. He did not move in, but he would spend the night with me, and I would allow him to drive my car. I was a huge step up for him, but he was a big step down for me. I think what really allowed me to be in this relationship was the fact that I felt it was all I had. I had spent so much time in isolation. I was extremely lonely and enjoyed the companionship. We began talking about marriage and everything. When I think about that now, that was extremely out of character. What was even crazier about this situation was that Rodney was the ex-boyfriend and child's father of one of the few friends that I was still connected to at this time, Natasha. Somehow Carmen, Rodney's sister, became aware of the relationship and threatened to tell Natasha, at least this is my recollection of it. Carmen has shared with me a different experience. Nevertheless, when it became apparent to me that someone else could tell Natasha that I was in a relationship with Rodney, I decided to tell her myself. I actually thought I was being mature in doing so. I cannot remember how she took it exactly, but by the next day, it was obvious that she was very hurt and angry. She removed me as her friend on Facebook and from what I remember was making posts about the situation. The news was spreading quickly. People were choosing sides, and mine was not the side they were choosing. I tried to spin the story to work in my favor, but that only gained a few supporters. I had known Rodney much longer than I had known Tasha. Besides, they were teenagers when they were together and had been separated for years. Looking back on this, that was a terrible thing to do; and although I do not use it as an excuse, I am well aware now that I was not in my right mind. My friend Terri was the only person who somewhat saw what was going on with me. I remember her meeting with me at Subway one day to try to get me to see my wrongdoing. Only, I was defensive and dismissive. In fact, others being against my relationship only fueled the fire and made me desire it even more because I was not going to allow anyone to tell me what I could and could not do. I even took Rodney home to meet my family. That is how invested I was. I am sure others saw that this was a mistake, but I think they were blaming me as a person of bad character, rather than as a person who was suffering from mental illness. Fortunately, the relationship did not last very long, no more than a few months. But the damage that it did would take years to heal. I became pregnant, and by this time, I was beginning to experience what most do after a hypomanic episode the polar opposite, another major depressive episode. It was as if someone had turned on the lights, and I was there left to look at all of the mess I had created. My depressive symptoms were really bad. I went back to my doctor to discuss resuming medication, but I was very confused about the different opinions of my doctor, my OB-GYN, and the pharmacist. One suggested I wait until the second trimester to return to taking the medication, for fear of what it would do to the unborn fetus. Another suggested the medication would not harm the baby at all and another suggested there was not enough evidence to demonstrate what kind of effect the medication could have on the fetus. I decided not to take the medication; although, I desperately needed it. Things began to get really bad again, but this time, I had no one to help me. The only person I had was Rodney, and he had no clue of what I was experiencing or the help that I needed. I was furious with him. Even though it takes a man and a woman to get pregnant, I know that he impregnated me intentionally. He thought that it would make me stay with him. I am not sure why he had not learned that this was not true, considering that he had five children by five different women. For a short while, I did feel stuck, and I felt even worse than I did before the hypomanic episode. I was working part-time and had enough income to cover my expenses, but I did not have any health insurance. I had not informed any of my providers that this was the case, and I continued seeing them as if I was covered. I figured I would continue until they found out. It got to the point where it was too difficult for me to even work. I went to the emergency room a few times. I had severe morning sickness that lasted all day. Looking back at it now, I am not sure if it was all morning sickness, or the depression, or the side effects from stopping the medication. I just know that I was sick, and I needed help desperately. My mother convinced me to do something I had sworn I would never do when I left to attend college, and that was to move back home. My brother Mark offered for me to stay with him in his apartment, and he lived very close to my mother. I resigned from my part-time teaching position, packed up my condo, and set out to leave. I actually abandoned it, because it still had not sold. It would not sell until the following August.

It was now December 2009. The year that had started out so hopeful with me pursuing a great dream had now turned into a nightmare. All that I had worked on and the reputation I had built for myself as a great school teacher and minister of the Gospel over the past eleven years had been destroyed in a matter of weeks. That's exactly what the enemy does. I would leave Fort Wayne now quietly and completely ashamed, returning to a place that had brought me so much hurt and disappointment as a child. I had no idea of how things would work out for me. In fact, I had lost all hope. I just knew that I could not stay where I was unless I wanted to die. I was pregnant, depressed, and alone. It could not get any worse than that.

CHAPTER 5

There Was A Glimpse of Hope

Things did not get better immediately once I returned home to my family, I had a few other challenges to overcome before I would be able to focus on my healing again. After visiting a clinic and hearing the abnormality of the fetus' heart rate and considering the possible side effects of taking the medication while pregnant, I decided to resume the medication because I was so low. Because of where I was at this point in my life, I decided to terminate the pregnancy. The idea of being forever linked to Rodney was too much to bear. It is not something that I am not proud of, but it is something I sought forgiveness for immediately and believe that God granted it. I felt instant remorse once it was over. I felt that my decision was influenced more by the opinions of others rather than my faith in God. Nevertheless, it was done, and there was nothing I could do but live with it. I went to church with my mother that Sunday, and when the Pastor called for people to come to the altar for prayer, I did. As I sat there, I remember praying, Lord, I need you to take this burden from me right now. I had known and heard of others who shared this experience talk about how it ate away at them and that it was something they never truly got over. I did not want that to be my experience. I wanted to receive forgiveness so that I could move on with my life. I knew that God had forgiven me, but now I was asking God to help me forgive myself, and He did precisely that. When I left that altar, I left that burden there, and it has never bothered me. I immediately started making plans to rebuild my life.

It was February of 2010 now, and I would soon be receiving my income tax refund. It would be a couple of thousands of dollars, enough to pay off some debt, pay some bills off, and do a few things I wanted to do, such as getting a gym membership. I had gained quite a bit of weight from the pregnancy, but more so from dealing with the depression. For nearly a year in Fort Wayne, I laid in the bed, and I comforted myself with food. A gas station with a Subway was right on the corner where I lived, and that is where I purchased food and snacks to eat. I wanted to begin exercising so I could begin losing the weight and feel better about myself again. On the morning my tax refund check hit my bank, I was extremely hopeful. I was up early checking my account balance, and once it hit, I hit the door. My first stop would be the license bureau to renew my license plates. When I got there, however, I was told I did not have the proper paperwork in order to change my address from Fort Wayne to Clarksville, Indiana. So, I left to retrieve what I needed and experienced something that would change my life forever. When I got out of the car, there was a small sheet of ice on the ground. However, I did not see it. Running to my brother's apartment to get my proper paperwork, I slipped and fell to the ground. Although I was in some pain, initially, I was not majorly concerned. I had fallen on ice years back when I lived in Fort Wayne. I once fell while walking to my car on my way to work. I fell backwards and hit my elbow. I thought I broke it while I laid there in pain, but after a few moments, I was able to shake it off. I thought this would be the case in this scenario as well. I thought I would lie there for a moment, and then get up and continue about my day. Only, when I went to get up, something felt extremely weird with my foot, or at least in that area. When I looked down, I realized I had dislocated my ankle. I could see my ankle bone through my sock. I was mortified. For a moment, I was helpless. Because I was only planning to briefly run into my brother's apartment to grab my paperwork for my license, I had left my cell phone in the car. It was early. I am not sure if it was even 9:00 am yet. I laid there on the cold ground before I decided to yell for help. Normally, my brother went to work early in the morning, but on this particular day for whatever reason, he was off. I yelled for a while before one of his neighbors finally came out. I cannot remember if my brother Mark finally heard me or if his neighbor went to get him, but he did eventually come. My brother tried to encourage me to get up and possibly hop on one leg so he could take me to the hospital, and I did try, but I simply could not. Finally, we called 9-1-1 to send an ambulance. His neighbor brought me a blanket while I waited. I am guessing Mark called my mother because she had arrived by this time as well. Once I got to the emergency room, and they did the X-rays, they found that my ankle was dislocated on one side and broken on both sides. Fortunately, an orthopedic surgeon had been at the hospital performing a surgery, and he decided that he would do mine as well. This was a tremendous blessing because at the time, I did not have any health insurance. This experience would cost me a lot physically and financially. I remember being in shock about what happened, and I needed a comfort that my family was not able to deliver. I remember asking the nurse to please find me a Gideon Bible, and I asked for my cell phone. I sent out a text message to different people in Fort Wayne asking them for prayer, and I held the Bible close to my chest while they took me back for surgery, I knew that my life would be forever changed, and it was.

The surgery went well, but my situation changed rather quickly. Now, instead of staying with Mark, I would have to stay with my mother. Mark lived on the third floor, and it was obvious that I would not be able to make it up the stairs. In fact, I had to stay an extra day at the hospital because I was not able to demonstrate using the crutches well. I had to use my oldest brother Junie's (Lowrence) walker instead. I did not want to stay with my mother. Too many people were already living there with her; Junie, my sister, and my two nephews. I really just wanted some distance and some privacy. Unfortunately, I did not have a choice. I went to stay with my mother, and I remained there for about two months before returning to stay with Mark. Being in my boot went from six weeks to nine weeks because I reinjured my ankle and had to have a second surgery to replace the plate. My mother had stairs as well, but she lived in a townhome. I slept on the couch and used the half bath to wash up. It was not completely unbearable, but there were days I just wanted some time to myself, and I could not get it.

There were two things that really helped me during this time, the library and my sister/friend, Mimi. I convinced my mother to take me to the library. I obtained a library card and started checking out books to read. Sometimes, I would have her just leave me at the library so I could have some time to myself. I remember one time sitting there while tears rolled down my face. I did not even try to conceal them. I had little strength to do so. I was overwhelmed being at my mother's house with my family. I had lived away from them for about fifteen years. I was used to living a certain way and in a totally different atmosphere. Reading different books was a tremendous help to me. It was an escape for me. I also read the Bible a lot, which strengthened my spirit. Mimi reached out to me and committed to being my prayer partner. We would connect every Thursday to have prayer together on the phone. I would go into the bathroom, and we would catch up with and pray for one another. I was seeking healing, employment, and a place of my own. It would be difficult to find a job, as most teaching positions only become available at the start of the school year. Staying with my mother and brother, I did not have a lot of bills, but I had some, and I needed income. My friend Michele joined me in prayer as well. Fortunately, she was now only an hour and a half away in Wilmore, Kentucky, and I was able to visit her as well. I decided to go into my retirement to help me until I was able to find another job. I was fortunate to find a full-time and a part-time teaching job, which was a tremendous blessing as I had acquired great debt from my ankle surgeries and the physical therapy that I needed in order to learn to walk on my own again. For an entire school year, I worked two jobs. I taught English at the high school I graduated from, Jeffersonville High School, and I taught as an adjunct instructor at Brown Mackie College, Louisville.

My brother decided he would downsize to a one bedroom apartment; so, this sped up my need to move out. I had wanted to save up a little more money before doing so, but I discerned that he was really ready to have his own place again. So, I found a one bedroom apartment in New Albany, Indiana. It was not far away, about fifteen minutes away maybe, but living in another city gave me the space I needed from my family. I was very thankful for my family and demonstrated that to them. That year, I made sure to buy all of my sibling's gifts for their birthday as a thank you for helping me during a very difficult time. I did not want to seem ungrateful. At the same time, I wanted to reestablish my independence apart from my family. It was something I had taken pride in for many years, and it was something I wanted to regain and did. I was not where I wanted to be, but I had determined to make the most of it. I was hopeful things would get better, and through prayer and much work, they did. I began exercising and following a new weight loss program, and I lost weight. I felt really good about myself. I was able to pay off a lot of my medical bills as well. An even greater blessing for me was Natasha and I had forgiven one another and moved forward in our friendship. In addition to Michele, she was now a trusted sister who would support me through the challenges I faced. In the midst of all of this, however, something else traumatic happened. My mother was diagnosed with endometrial cancer. This was in 2011. I stood right by her side through the hospital stays and all, and I saw my mother fight and kick cancer's butt. She made it look so easy, that in 2013 when I got the chance to leave, I took it without any hesitation.

In 2012, we lost my brother, Junie. He had a brain aneurysm and died instantly. I remember getting the phone call at work. I cannot remember if it was the assistant principal or the school secretary who called and told me I had a phone call downstairs. I immediately knew that it was bad news. The only other time I had gotten called to the office like this was when my grandmother had died, my father's mother. Then, my mother shared it with my principal, and he told me. Due to previous experiences, I had conversations with my mother and told her to never call me (again) in a hysteria, that there was a way to inform people of tragic events. For a while, I avoided the call. I did not want to hear the news that would be coming from the other end. I did eventually go downstairs and found it was my mother calling. She told me that my brother had a brain aneurysm, that it was not looking good, and that I needed to get to the hospital when I could. Somehow, I did not believe her. It was not that I did not believe that the situation was happening, but in my heart, I knew that my brother Junie was already gone and that they were just waiting for me to get there to tell me the bad news. I took my time leaving work that day. I did not leave immediately. I finished out the school day, and I stayed to leave lesson plans for the remainder of the week. I believe this all occurred on a Wednesday, so I left plans for Thursday and Friday. When I got to the hospital, Junie was on a respirator. My other siblings had left, but I had heard about the drama that took place. I was told that when they told my mother about his condition and she broke down, that my second oldest brother Michael began verbally attacking her asking her why she was upset because she knew this was going to happen and that he blamed her. Junie was an alcoholic. He lived with my mother. But although she may have known more about his behaviors and health than we did, she was certainly not responsible for his death.

When I arrived, things were calm. I remember my sister coming in to kiss Junie goodbye once she realized we were going to take him off the machine. She was not in agreement. Nevertheless, once I arrived and saw the situation, I knew it was something that had to be done, and I supported my mother through that. Looking back at things now, in addition to my mother overcoming cancer and losing her oldest son, perhaps I should not have left when I did to move to Arizona, but I was truly trying to save my own life. We ended up burying my brother, Junie, or should I say that I did. My mother was convinced he had life insurance, but he did not. He had only been paying on a term life insurance policy for a few months, and so it was no good. No one else offered to pay anything, and looking back at it now, I wish I had not, or at least not to the degree that I did. I wish I would have taken more time to research our options and taken the least costly one. I did not want to see my mother made ashamed, so I offered my credit card to pay for the funeral expenses, which was a little over five thousand dollars. My mother and my siblings agreed that they would help me to pay it off, but they did not. I believe the amount I asked for was about thirty dollars a month. While I still lived there, they paid me, but when I moved to Arizona, everyone, except for Mark, seemed to not know how to get the money to me. I was left with the balance of the bill. This was a great hardship for a few reasons. One because a few months after Junie died, my engine died, and I had to get a new car with a car payment, and my income decreased when I moved to Arizona. They never tried to make it right, nor did they ever even apologize. I am not sure if they ever even thanked me. I loved Junie; he was my oldest brother, but I did not do what I did for him, I did it for my mother. Junie was twenty-three years older than me. We did not grow up together, and we were not really close. He was more of an authoritative figure in my life growing up. He was who my mother called when my older siblings were getting out of hand. Towards the end of his life however, he succumbed to his drug and alcohol addiction. He developed cirrhosis of the liver and other health problems, and my mother took care of him. During the few months I lived with my mother, and he lived there as well, I was able to spend a little more time with him, and I was glad for that.

When I first came home from the hospital after having surgery, he helped me when I would have to get up from the couch. When I wanted to go to church, even though he did not go to church, he went so he could help push me in the wheelchair. He did what he could to play the role of my oldest brother, and I was thankful for that. He worked a part-time job at Kroger, and one year, they were selling Snuggies. I think that is what they were called. They are like small throw blankets that have a hoodie on them. I wanted one so bad, and he had my mother buy one and give it to me for my birthday. It is the only thing I have of him. My older siblings took everything out of his room right after he died. They did not consult my mother or anyone else. By the time they were done going through his things, it was as if he had never even lived there. They took everything.

It was during this time that I visited my doctor to resume taking my medication and sought out a new therapist. I felt myself going down and I knew I needed to be stable in order to stand with my mother. After Junie died, it seemed like there was one event after the other. Michael and Derek were hospitalized; and both for similar things. They were both addicts as well. Michael had overcome his drug use for many years, but for whatever reason, he started using again. This was extremely disheartening because Michael and I had grown closer over the years. He was the sibling I disliked the most as a child. He was mean and always in a bad mood. When his girlfriend died, when I was seventeen years old, he turned his life around. He stopped drinking and using drugs. He started going to church and eventually, he found a good woman, and he married her. I accepted my calling to preach the Gospel and had preached at my mother's church. As a gift to me, Michael gave me his father's gold necklace that had a cross. He wanted me to wear it when I preached so that he felt like a part of him and his father were with me. After that, Michael and I started getting closer. I would visit him when I came home, and once I moved home, I would visit him a lot. We would talk about different things that we did not like concerning the family, and we would both try to do things that made our mother happy. However, that all changed once he started hanging out with our brother Derek again.

One night, I walked into a situation in which he appeared to be having a nervous breakdown. He was screaming and yelling at his wife. I did not know what to do, so I called my mother. That was a crazy night. I still am not sure what completely happened to set him off. I believe his wife knew what he was doing with Derek and that she was trying to get him to stop, and he became angry. Junie and my sister said that he was on some type of drugs. After Junie died and he ended up in the hospital, it was something that was going on with his heart. I was told that he had been trying to use drugs again with Derek and that it affected his heart. I cannot remember what caused Derek to end up in the hospital, but I do remember that he almost died. He was on life support and everything. I just know that it was too much and that I did not want to stay here. When I would follow-up with my doctor, I would share with her the different events going on in my family. One time, I remember her saying that I did not need medicine but that I just needed to get away from my family. I agreed with her, and that was what I set in my heart to do.

Initially, I considered moving to Nashville, Tennessee. My friend Natasha was wanting to move at that time too, and she had asked if I would consider Nashville. Nashville was only about three hours away, close enough if anything happened, but far enough to live my own life separate from the chaos of my family. I had gone back to being that little girl who was always nervous when the phone rang. Because you never knew the news you would get on the other end and my mother would try to guilt me into supporting my older siblings no matter what. "That's your brother", she would say. "You do not kick a person when they are down", she would say. But I knew that if I kept getting wrapped up in their lives that I would never have a life of my own. This is not what I wanted. This was not what I had fought for as a child or how I had managed to live my life the fifteen years I was away from them. I was not like them, and I did not want to be associated with them. I wanted to be my own person. I wanted out.

When the opportunity came for me to move to Arizona, I took it. I also had another opportunity in Memphis, Tennessee, but Arizona seemed to be the better option. My sorority sister, Kim, lived there. We had both lived in Fort Wayne for many years and she was a big help to me. It was through her that I developed a closer relationship with the Lord and recognized the calling on my life, and she had helped me on one occasion with my weight loss. By this time, I had gained back the thirty pounds I had lost plus some, and things did not seem they would be any better. So, even though I knew that some did not understand, I left. It was the glimpse of hope I needed to rebuild my life. I did not leave intending to stay gone forever. I just wanted enough time to get back to being the strong person I once was and knew I was at my core. I knew I could not do that surrounded by dysfunction and turmoil. Within a matter of weeks, I had packed up my apartment, mapped out my travel, and was off to the west coast.

CHAPTER 6

This Was Not What I Expected

When I first arrived in Arizona, I was so hopeful. I was finally away from what I thought brought me low, my family. Let me clarify that when I speak of the negativity of my family that I am speaking of my immediate family, mainly my older brothers and sister. I was reunited with my sorority sister, Kim, again, and it felt so good. In my mind, I was really going to thrive here. I was going to get back to being the 'Chelle-B. that I used to be and loved. I initially stayed with Kim and her then husband and youngest daughter until I found an apartment of my own, which was a little bit more challenging than I had imagined. Kim lived in Phoenix, but I would be working in Queen Creek, which was about a forty-five-minute drive. Considering that I had taken an almost ten thousand dollar pay cut, I knew I did not want to have that long of a commute in which I would be spending a lot more on gas. I searched for an entire month in various surrounding cities. Finally, I contacted an apartment finder agency who was able to help me locate an apartment in Mesa. Mesa was in between Phoenix and Queen Creek, which I thought would be perfect. I tried to stay around the same amount that I was paying for rent in Indiana, but the apartment I found cost a little more. I wanted to live where I would be comfortable. I tried to stay away from anywhere that had an infestation of scorpions and other critters.

A few months before leaving Indiana, the water heater in my apartment had gone out and caused a flood in my apartment that ruined my furniture. From that claim, I was able to relocate to Arizona and buy new furniture. I had only brought things that could fit in my car, such as clothing, dishes, my flat screen television, and other small odds and ends. I bought a really nice living room and bedroom set at a store during their Fourth of July sale. I arrived in Arizona on the Fourth of July. I considered it to be my personal independence day. Along with the dining table that Kim gifted me and a few other household items and décor, I would be set. I immediately began training for my new teaching position which would be my first experience at a charter school. Training lasted for two weeks. It was so much information to learn. I am not sure what I retained, but I was excited to be there. This school would be a very different experience for me. Unlike the other two schools I had taught at it was predominately white. In addition, most of the students and staff were of the Mormon faith. It took some adjusting, but it turned out to be one of the best experiences I had ever had. Many of my students had never engaged with a Black person before. Some even told me that I was the first relationship they had ever shared with a Black person. I was only there for two years, but by the time I left, I had students calling me Mom and Auntie just as I had at my other schools by my Black students.

My school required a lot of me; I worked harder there than I have at any other teaching assignment, and for less pay. The workday was longer. We were required to submit lesson plans for the entire year at the start of the school year. As an English teacher, I was required to assign a major essay each quarter. We were required to do after school tutoring and contact parents weekly. It was a lot. I had more students than I had ever had before, over two hundred. We were on block scheduling so, I had to plan longer lesson plans, and I would only have a planning period every other day. It was a lot. Some days, I would be so tired that all I could do was go home and get into bed so I could prepare to do it all over again the next day. I would endure headaches from all of the grading I had to do. One night, I ended up in the emergency room due to a migraine I acquired while grading. I hated essay time. It would take days for me to grade all of the essays. And yet, I had some of the best relationships with my students than I ever had. Unlike my other schools, I was able to discipline my students when they did not complete their assignments. After so many missed assignments, I was able to assign them detention to complete the work, and if they did not attend detention, they could be suspended. The dean of students was amazing. I held my students accountable, and he backed me up every time. Parents were actually concerned and involved in their students' education. They would call, come to conferences, and observe their students' progress online. This was never my experience prior to this school.

When it became known that my mother was ill and even after her death, some of my students were so supportive. I had a few students who served as assistants who would do some of my grading, create my bulletin boards, and make most of my copies. They were such a blessing. I would not have made it without them, and I was sure to thank them with random gifts throughout the year. I would receive flowers, cards, and other special notes from my students. They encouraged me so much. I would not have made it through in the strength that I did without them. Although school was a successful experience, I was frustrated with the amount of my time it consumed. I felt like I did not have time for a personal life outside of school. I came to Arizona with the mindset that my sorority sister Kim was already plugged into the church and social life and that through her, I would be able to do the same. However, I soon learned that was not the case. In her defense, she worked for the same district as I did as a principal, and her job was very demanding. She was also in a marriage in which she did not have fulfillment. I am happy to report that she is now in a very thriving marriage, working for a different district, and in a much better place than she was when I lived there. I thought we would do the things we had done together in Fort Wayne years ago, such as go to church together and exercise together, but we did not. I became extremely angry and frustrated with her. It was not until later that I realized that these were unfair expectations I had placed upon her. My leading a better life was not dependent upon her or anyone else. It was up to me to make my life better.

At the end of my first school year there, I sadly learned that my mother's cancer had returned; only this time, it was terminal. I was devastated and confused. How could she be terminal when she had just received a clean bill of health that January, and this was only April or May? I did not understand that at all. I still don't, and I imagine I never will. Nevertheless, I knew I had to get home to my mother. I had seen her when I went to visit during my Christmas break, and she appeared to be well. I was not sure if I would be going just for the summer or if I would be moving back permanently.

I had just signed a contract with my district which they had just initiated. The contract agreement was that if I resigned from my position before the end of the next school year that I would have to pay a two-thousand dollar fine. In addition, I was still under my apartment lease and if I broke it, I would have to pay a fifteen hundred dollar fine and there were no exceptions. I bought a one-way ticket back home and packed what I could. When I got home, my mother was staying with my sister in her apartment, which I did not like. I did not understand why she could not have just stayed with my mother so that she could remain in an environment that was familiar to her. My sister lived in a tower apartment building that was for lower income adults. The apartments had been nice when I was a child, but they were now extremely run down. My sister said it was easier for her to take care of her small apartment than my mother's three-bedroom townhome. I think she also did not want to be at my mother's because that is where our oldest brother had died. Still, she had only lived in her own apartment for a few months, and I thought that was extremely selfish. She had rarely ever had a place of her own. She had always lived with my mother and now when my mother needed her, she chose to put herself before my mother, and I was not happy about that. When I walked in the door and saw my mother on the couch, I was shocked. She looked so sick and was so weak. She was in a lot of pain. She burst into tears when she saw me, as if she knew she would finally be okay. I called her doctor immediately and convinced my mother to go to the hospital as her doctor had recommended. I stayed with her at the hospital just as I had done when she was initially treated for the cancer three years prior. To my understanding, the cancer had spread to her lungs and elsewhere. She was spitting up blood. She had decided to take chemotherapy again, and it was a very strong dosage. When the oncologist came to see her, my mother told me she wanted to know how long she had left to live. I talked to Dr. Parker, and she explained to me that with treatment, she may extend her life about six months, but that the quality of her life would be poor. She would rather my mother not do the treatment, but then, she would maybe live another month. My mother decided to continue the treatment. There were two things she desperately wanted to live to see, my brother Mark get married, and her first great-grandchild. And fortunately, she did live to see both. When it came time for my mother to be discharged from the hospital, it was recommended that she go to a rehab facility before returning home. She had lost her ability to walk, and I knew she did not want that. She wanted to be able to walk down the aisle at my brother's wedding, not be pushed in a wheelchair. Initially, she did not want to go, but I convinced her by telling her that we would find a nice facility and that I would stay with her while she was there. She agreed to go and was able to regain her strength and ability to walk after about twenty-one days there. I was there with her the entire summer. It was extremely frustrating dealing with my older siblings because of their lack of involvement. I would ask them to come sit with her long enough so that I could look for a job, but they never did. If they came, they always came in the evening and would only stay briefly. One time, when I got my oldest living sibling, Michael, to come sit with her, he called me multiple times in the brief time that I was away. He wanted me to return so that he could tend to something at his house. I am not sure what they thought was going to happen. Maybe they thought I could just make a phone call and get a job, but it was not that easy. I was not going to leave my job in Arizona without having a new job, especially since it would cost me over three thousand dollars to break my work contract and my apartment lease. My older siblings wanted me to do everything, which I felt was extremely unfair. At one point, Michael actually used the term Messiah when referring to me because he said I had come to save our mother and save them.

I think I accepted sooner than others that my mother was going to die and that there was nothing even I could do about that. When I brought my mother home from rehab, it turned into even greater turmoil. While I was out picking up her prescription, Michael and my sister, Shellie, came to get her. I was extremely upset. They did not consult me or any of the rest of us. They had not been there at all for her while she was in the hospital or rehab, and now here they were trying to take over. Yet, they wanted me to stay and do everything. I decided then I would go back to Arizona. I found myself a one-way ticket back, and as hard as it was for me to leave my mother, I did. Things would be even harder in Arizona for me now with me having to work and worry about my mother back home. I called frequently and flew back home once or twice a month between August and when she died in December. I tried to make things better for myself in Arizona. I decided I would stop depending on Kim to help move my life forward, and I began doing things. I found a church. I became active in my sorority. I began accepting invitations from a sister I had met and I began to be more social.

My mother was able to walk down the aisle at my brother's wedding, and she saw my great-nephew, Aydin, when he was a few weeks old. Thanksgiving was my last real time with her. We were all together at my sister's, my siblings, nephews, nieces, and I. It was so hard for me to be there with my mother and not lose it dealing with my sister. My sister had grown tired of taking care of her and told Michael and I that after Christmas she would have to go. She was mean to my mother. She was taking money from her account without her permission. I knew this because I had access to my mother's account. She was the last place I would want my mother to be. I held my tongue many days out of respect for my mother, and because I was somewhat at her mercy. I did not live there, and I knew I was not the one caring for her twenty-four seven at this time. That would be the last time I saw my mother sitting up and talking, although she was extremely tired at that time. After that visit, I decided I did not want my mother living with my sister anymore. My assistant principal had talked with the board to see if I could get out of my contract without penalty, and when I renewed my apartment lease, I only did a six month lease, instead of twelve. My lease would now end in February instead of August. The plan was for me to teach through Dr. Martin Luther King Day at the end of January. I would pay February's rent at the end of January with my last check, and I would move home to take care of my mother. I would move her to Michael's home. I put in an application to return to my part-time teaching position at Brown Mackie College, Louisville. I felt myself going down, and I also felt the heavy burden of what was ahead of me. I resumed taking my antidepressant, and it was really good that I did because my plans to return home would happen sooner than I had planned.

In December, a week before my Christmas break, I received a call that my mother had been taken to the hospital and that things were not looking good. I only had a few sick days remaining, but I knew I could not wait. I decided to return home to be with my mother. I missed out on a week and half of pay, but I needed to be there with her. I was getting most of my information from Michael, and I had learned that he was not giving me true information. He was in denial about my mother's illness and was not accepting that she was going to die. He had told me over the phone that the doctors had said that my mother's problem was that she was not eating. He said they wanted to give her a feeding tube, send her to rehab again, and that she would be okay. That did not sound right to me. I also knew my mother never wanted a feeding tube. She did not want to be resuscitated either. I took a flight and made it to my mother's hospital room at night. When I got there, no one was there. I was told by my aunt that they had told my mother earlier that morning there was nothing else medically they could do for her and that my siblings left after receiving this news. I was furious to find her alone. I stayed the night with her, and the next day, met with someone from hospice. My brother Mark and I made the necessary decision to move her to inpatient hospice care where she would receive the care she needed to be made comfortable. I spent eight days with my mother there, and on the eighth day, while my brother, his wife, and I sang hymns to her, she peacefully departed from this world. It was as if I did not have time to grieve because I had to comfort everyone else. I was the minister in the family and the one who my mother had left in charge of her affairs. I had to plan her funeral. I included my siblings in all of the planning. I did not want anyone to say I took over. I made sure we did everything my mother had asked, the color she wanted to wear and for her casket, who she wanted listed in her obituary, the songs she wanted to be sung. My older siblings wanted me to speak, and I did that as well. It was one of the hardest things I have ever had to do. Without God and without being back on my antidepressant, there is no way I would have been able to make it through any of that.

When everything was over and I returned to Arizona, things became even more difficult for me. I thought I would have more support from my sorority sister Kim, but I did not. I was not sure why. Maybe she was dealing with her own problems. Maybe she did not realize my pain. Maybe she had felt the frustration I had felt toward her prior to my mother's death. Nevertheless, I needed someone, and no one was there. Because I had not lived in Arizona that long and because I was spending most of my weekends traveling home to be with my mother, I had not really developed any strong relationships, not even within my church. For months, I simply went to work and came home and got in the bed. I longed for someone, anyone, back home to come see about me, but no one ever did. I isolated myself more and more. I deactivated my Facebook page. I did not want to talk to anyone. I had nothing good to say. After a few months, I decided that enough was enough, and that because no one was coming to save me, I had to save myself. I resumed the things I had started doing before my mother's death while in Arizona. I started going back to church. I started attending sorority meetings. I started connecting with some of the ladies I had met, and I started attending more social events. There was a comedy club in Phoenix I would go to on the weekends. Those comedy shows gave me so much laughter and life. Laughter truly is like medicine and good for the soul, and those shows helped me tremendously. I even went to the comedy club in Tempe. I saw comedians such as Rickey Smiley, Simmore, Gary Owens, Charlie Murphy, Bruce Bruce, Lavelle Crawford, and Deon Cole. They were all amazing. I continued to take my medication also. I am not sure why I never pursued a therapist while living there. I did attend a group therapy that focused on grief and loss. After a few sessions, however, I stopped attending. The group had grown enormously large, and I did not feel that it gave the help I needed individually. So, I just fought through it all on my own. By the end of the school year, I had decided I needed my support system back home. I decided not to renew my teaching contract nor my apartment lease. I would be leaving without having a job back home, but I was hopeful I would gain employment. I just strongly felt that if I stayed in Arizona, I would not have the support I needed to regain my strength permanently. It was not what I thought it was going to be, and I did not want to stay.

The last month there, I sold my furniture, shipped my clothes back home, and moved into a studio apartment. It was a very pleasant experience. I wished I had found it before moving into my other apartment. It was furnished, and it included utilities and the internet. It had a fitness and laundry room. It was clean, quiet, and safe. Had I stayed there first, I would have had more time to decide if I really wanted to stay in Arizona before buying furniture and making it a home, and I would have had more time to choose a better place to live. To help me make the drive back, my friend and sister, Natasha, flew to Arizona. That was such a blessing for her to help me through that, not only the drive, but the sadness I felt in leaving Arizona and going back home to the unknown. The last few days of the school year were difficult because I was saying goodbye to students and families I had grown to love. A few days before I left, I met two of my female students and their moms for lunch. I called them my daughter and my niece, even though they were white. We exchanged gifts and laughter and lots of love and tears. As I share this now, it makes me a little sad. Unlike my other teaching jobs that I had left, I knew I would probably never see these girls again. Thank goodness for social media. One of them I am still able to follow. The other one is not really on there as much. But, through social media, I have been able to remain connected to many of my students, and that has been a tremendous blessing.

Arizona was not at all what I had expected. There was some good and some bad. I had no idea I would lose my mother in such a short time but, I remember the prayer she prayed over me the day when I left. In her prayer, she said she knew I belonged to God and that He would take care of me. Those words would be just as true the day I left to move to Arizona as the day I left to move back home. I would face many challenges, but God would take care of me.

CHAPTER 7

Things Got Worse

The trip to return home was not as exciting as the trip to Arizona. On the road to Arizona, I was full of hope about my future. On the road leaving Arizona, however, I was full of uncertainty and even some fear. My mother had died, and my brother Mark had gotten married. I did not have a home to return to. I also did not have job security. I had the money from selling my furniture and a few more checks from the school year. I would be home for a few months before I would secure a job and my own apartment. In the meantime, I visited with friends in various cities, Fort Wayne, Indiana, Chicago, Illinois, and Lexington, Kentucky. I stayed a few nights with my brother, but I never stayed long. I did not want to be a burden, especially since he was newly married. I would try to only stay with him when I was looking for a job. I decided to apply for a teaching job in Louisville, Kentucky; rather than going back to Jeffersonville, Indiana. My Indiana license had expired, and so getting a job in Louisville would be much easier; plus, I would make more money. I must add that I did not leave Jeffersonville High School on a good note. The principal, who had been assistant principal when I was there, did not see eye to eye when it came to disciplining a particular student. This student was a girl, and she was terrible. She was a huge behavior problem. I knew it was due to her poor academics, but she would not allow me to help her. Instead, she would be defiant and downright disrespectful, which I did not tolerate. The assistant principal turned principal had asked me to not remove her from the classroom and to work with her due to her home life experience, and I tried to do that, but she would just go too far, and I would have to send her out. I could not allow her too openly be disrespectful towards me. I also had twenty plus other students I needed to teach who were willing to learn. I have always shared the philosophy of never allowing one or a few students to completely disrupt the learning process for all. I remember the assistant principal now principal sending me an email in which she demonstrated her disagreement and disappointment with me, and she copied it to the other assistant principals and the principal I believe. I responded to her via email and by showing up at her office. I do not tolerate disrespect from adults either, even if they are my superior. I am never nasty or rude, but I will defend myself and my position, and that is what I did. Even with that, I do know that my leaving to go to Arizona was felt. When I reported to Human Resources to turn in my resignation, because it was summertime, the lady who had hired me told me that the assistant principal now principal spoke of my leaving and the high test scores that my students had that year. My students had one of the highest, if not the highest state standardized test scores in the building. One thing no one would ever say about me was that I was not a good teacher because I knew I was.

My brother Mark was now living in Louisville with his wife, and so I preferred to live there as well. It was more challenging getting a job in the Louisville school system. Unlike Indiana and Arizona where I was able to directly apply to the school in which I wanted to teach, I had to apply to the district and let them make my assignment based on how they saw fit. Because of my years of experience and my master's level degree, based on my conversation with my cousin who had retired from the district, I knew I would be assigned to a low performing school. Although I did not want that, I was desperate. I knew that even though I had taught for fifteen years and had proven myself elsewhere that was not the case here. Here, I would have to start over and prove myself all over again. The summer was quickly going by, and I was becoming extremely impatient. I came up with a strategy to mail my resume to particular schools in hopes that they would reach the principals directly and my strategy worked. My resume reached a principal who was in need of an English teacher. I was licensed to teach speech and theatre arts as well, but English was my primary subject. I attended the interview and was offered the job. I wanted to wait for other opportunities, but there did not appear to be any, so I took it. I did not feel good about the assignment at all, but at least it was a job, and I was able to get my own apartment, which I found a few miles away from the school and away from where my brother Mark lived.

I did my best to settle into the new job assignment. I set up my classroom, and I attended the opening days. But, in that short time span, I felt an anxiety that I had never experienced before. I was so anxious I was nauseous. I could not focus during any of the training sessions. Everything presented seemed extremely overwhelming to me. At home, I was still extremely anxious. All I wanted to do was sleep, but I could not. I called to get my antidepressant medication refilled only to realize that was a mistake. When I was taking them in Arizona, I had gradually increased to a higher dosage, but as I had done in the past, I stopped taking it abruptly. So, when I resumed taking the medication, I should have done so at the lower dose, but I did with the higher dose. I found myself being even more anxious and reached out to the pharmacist to see what I could do to calm it down and to get some sleep. He said I could take Benadryl. I took it about every four hours. I would take it, fall asleep, wake up, and then take it again to go back to sleep. I did this for an entire weekend. By this time, I was in my new apartment, and I had purchased some furniture and some things I needed. I did not know why, but I felt extremely intimidated by this position. I felt incompetent. I was working with another teacher who was new. Her classroom was super decorated, and she had already started planning out her lessons. I did not even know where to begin. I met with my cousin Emma who tried her best to encourage me. I even called the Pastor whom I had the inappropriate relationship with. I had not spoken with him in years, but I was desperate, and he was someone from my past who I could go to for counsel and support. I remember telling him I was not going to be able to do it and him telling me that I could. While sitting in a training, I remember having an anxiety attack. I absolutely could not catch my breath. I stepped outside. I cannot remember completely how it happened, but I believe I called my cousin Emma and explained to her what I was experiencing. She told me to go talk to Human Resources. At first, I did not feel they could help me as I had technically not even begun teaching. I had only been hired a few days before school started, set up my classroom, and attended two days of training. Fortunately, those two days was all I needed to essentially be employed. When I got to the district office and went to see HR, there was a Black woman working there. I am sure she must have seen the panic on my face as she told me to come in and close the door. She asked me what was wrong. I told her I had just moved back here, I had lost my mother, and I was dealing with some extreme anxiety and did not think I could do the job. She explained to me about FMLA and told me I needed to see my doctor immediately. Fortunately, I was able to contact the doctor I had before moving to Arizona, and she agreed to see me that afternoon. I went to her office, explained to her what was going on with me, and was able to get her to sign off on my FMLA. I took it back to the district, and it was approved. I was relieved. I would be able to take up to twelve weeks off. I would not receive any payment, but I would have some time, and that is what I felt I needed. The hard part would be telling my new boss and telling my brother Mark. My boss was very confused, and I am sure pretty stressed; for school would be starting the next week, and he was now without a teacher. I am not completely sure how Mark felt about my decision, but I know he felt the burden of now having to worry about me, not only mentally but financially as well. He did go up to the building with me to take down my classroom. I knew in my heart I would not be returning to that school. I cannot explain the feeling I would get when I entered that building, but it was not good at all. The goal would be for me to hopefully receive another teaching assignment at a different school. In order to do that, however, I had to give up my current assignment. This was very scary as there was no guarantee a position would become available after the school year had already started.

I did give up my assignment. I then became a teacher without an assignment, and there was nothing I could do but pray and patiently wait for God to intervene. I rested a lot and gave my medicine time to work. In about a month, I felt better and was ready to go back to work. I received a call about another assignment at a different school. It was not extremely better than the other teaching assignment, but it was much better, and I felt more at ease about it. I was hired for the job, and I was extremely grateful to God. It was a bit challenging at first. I was taking over classrooms that had been led by a permanent substitute, an attractive young Black male at that. Some of my students resisted, and it took a while for all of us to adjust, but we did eventually. I do not remember exactly when it started, but I began to feel depressed again. I continued with medication off and on, and I began seeing the therapist again whom I had been with before moving to Arizona. Towards the end of the school year, she recommended me receiving treatment through an outpatient program at a behavioral hospital. She believed it would help provide me with some support as well as structure during the time I would be off work. By this time, my anxiety had turned to depression, and I was pretty deep in it. I would experience severe fatigue. I would have little strength or desire to do anything. I agreed to the outpatient program. It was somewhat helpful, but it was not completely helpful. My insurance would cover four weeks, five days a week, for about four to five hours a day. I was assigned to an all female group. For the first three hours, I would be in that group. Then, we would have lunch followed by another hour of group therapy. The second group therapy was coed and was compiled of people from various other groups. Every so often, I would meet with a psychiatrist to discuss medication. I never met with them for any length of time, and I never felt that the medication really helped me. I continued to feel exhausted and lacked very little strength or desire to do anything once I left each day. The women's group therapy I did not feel was beneficial to me. The majority of the women in the group were dealing with domestic abuse and drug addiction, neither of which was my experience. I only remember the therapist addressing me and my concerns once the entire time I was there. She told me I was dealing with codependency. I did not see it at the time; she did not really help me to see it, but I did much later. I spent most of my time there listening to the other women share about their relationship and drug related experiences. The coed group was not beneficial at all. Looking back at it now, it seems we did some sort of play therapy, such as coloring. I had no idea how coloring was going to help me, and it did not. I attended much of the program, but I did not finish my entire time. Patients were only allowed to miss so much time, and I had exceeded my time. There were days I would wake up, and I just could not find the strength to even put clothes on to attend, and so I did not. This was the summer of 2016.

Summer would end and a new school year would begin. I am not sure why, but as time went on, starting a new school year became more and more stressful for me. I would become extremely depressed as the beginning of a new school year approached. In fact, I would dread it. I hated starting over. I was not one of those teachers who did a lot of reading and planning and attending professional development in preparation for the new school year during the summer. By this time, teaching no longer served as a passion for me. It had become a job. It was what I knew how to do and what I did to earn a living. Once I got back to the building, however, I would be fine. I would get back into the routine. I would set up my classroom and I would get back to work. My episodes of depression would be off and on throughout the school year. As time went on, it seemed to be more on than off. It would seem that I would only have a few good months before the depression would return and consume my very being. More symptoms were appearing now. In addition to the fatigue, I would experience feeling extremely overwhelmed. Things and situations that would have normally been minor became super gigantic and difficult to manage. I began to lose confidence in myself and my abilities more and more. I felt like I was merely surviving but not doing a very good job of it. I was less engaged with my family, but they were still there with their dysfunction. By this time, I had begun setting some boundaries and distancing myself.

Things were never really the same after my mother died. I was angry with them, but doing my best not to cut all ties, even though that is what I wanted to do. Mark still had a relationship with them, and so in a sense, I felt I was supposed to. I was angry with them because they never repaid me for burying our older brother who died with no insurance, and they never repaid me for covering the headstone for our mother. Mark was the only one who did. He even tried to compensate for some of their part, which I thought was unfair. The only time I was around them was during the holidays, but even that had begun to subside. In 2017, I started the year out strong. In February of that year, during Black History month, my Pastor had preached a sermon about Fences. He had gotten the title from a very popular movie that was out, starring Denzel Washington and Viola Davis. In his sermon, he taught about the purpose and the value of fences or creating boundaries, and I identified with a lot of it. I decided that was what I was going to do with some of the relationships in my life, particularly with my older siblings and a few of my so-called friends. I began distancing myself and speaking my mind a lot more, something I never did before. My siblings were so much older than me, so I never felt allowed to say what I really wanted to say to them.

My sister was extremely violent, and she used fear as her tactic to have her way. By this time, the drugs and alcohol slowed her down. She and Michael would call me about my nephew's daughter and their frustration with her mother. They were so critical of her and always had something negative to say against her. They would call me trying to get me to go to the courthouse against her, and when I refused, they became very angry with me. They knew they could not do it because they did not know what to say or whom to speak with about their complaints. They had always been so dependent on my mother. They were trying to make me take on my mother's role, and I refused, which infuriated them even more. At one point, I blocked them from even being able to contact me. This was after we were supposed to meet at Michael's one day to go through some boxes containing my mother's belongings. It had been three years since she passed, and he still had everything and was not intending to share anything. He just took over, as he did after our oldest brother died. I am not sure why he felt so entitled, but he did. When we all met up at his house and began to look through things, Mark and I quickly realized that they had already taken everything and that what was left were items that had been destroyed. It was basically trash. It was at that point I decided I was done with them. I had endured years of my childhood suffering due to them. I was an adult now, Mama was gone, and I no longer had to put up with it. I built a fence, and I have never regretted it. I began to focus more on myself and decided I would finally return to school to pursue something else. I had wanted to leave teaching for a long time. I just did not know what it was that I would do. I thought it was attending seminary to become a Pastor, but that plan did not work out.

I realized that in dealing with my own battles with mental health that I could serve as a licensed therapist. I wanted to be the help I received, but I also wanted to be the help that I never received. I was still up and down with my depression and was very fearful about my ability to finish school, but I had to do something if I was ever going to move forward. I had finally found a psychiatrist at this time, and sometimes the medicine would seem to work. I was very hopeful about attending school. It would not be my first choice, which was to pursue Marriage and Family Therapy at Louisville Presbyterian Theological Seminary, but it would be a close second. I would pursue a Master of Science in Social Work at the University of Louisville. I chose MSSW and U of L over MAFT and LPTS because LPTS did not have evening classes. At the time, my therapist was encouraging me to walk away from teaching and to pursue the MAFT at LPTS, but I did not see how that was possible. They had scholarships to cover tuition, but how would I live? She had a husband who had a very good job, and so she could not identify with my challenge. So, I decided to go to U of L. I wanted to do the two-year program, but that would have been too much, so I did the three-year program.

In the three-year program, I would not begin my practicum experience until the second year. This would give me an opportunity to learn to manage being back in school and teaching full-time. I would take two classes per semester, including the summer. I started off doing very well. I was not completely fond of my Social Policy course, but I was very intrigued with my Human Behavior course. The first several weeks of the course, my professor would have us to keep a daily journal. She would give us certain questions or topics to consider. When we returned to class, we would spend the first part sharing what we had written. It was like going to therapy for me. I absolutely loved it, and

I thrived. I did a really good job of balancing school, work, and even my personal life. I was not overwhelmed. I would take it one semester at a time, and I knew I would succeed. Things were going very well until they weren't. My sister would die at the end of my first semester, and even though we were not super close, and I did not feel any major grief, what I would experience during this time would rattle my entire world.

CHAPTER 8

I Would Have Never Imagined Things Like This

When my sister died, I had no intentions of being involved in her funeral arrangements. My brother Mark and I had been called to the hospital a few days before she passed. Michael had told our Auntie Shirley to call and tell us we needed to get there. However, when we got there and found him and Derek in the room with her, they shared nothing with us. We were not even sure why they had called since we both had visited with her earlier that day. Much like with my mother, I knew that my sister was dying perhaps before others. Maybe they knew too, but they just did not want to accept it. The previous spring when she was in the hospital, I took off work a few times to be with her and to meet with the doctors directly, something that my older siblings did not understand you needed to do in order to truly know what was going on. She had been diagnosed with diabetes, but the doctors were looking for something else as well; cancer. My sister said she did not want to know if she had cancer. I believe she already knew.

I tried to be there for her. I visited her. I took her sugar-free treats. But when I would think about all she had done, it became extremely difficult for me to stand with her. When she got out of the hospital. Things went back to the way they had been with them and their drama, and I distanced myself. I did mention to Michael that they needed to make sure her insurance payments were up-to-date. In September of that year, 2017, I received a call from Derek telling me Shellie was really sick and that they could not get her to go to the hospital. As usual, they wanted me to intervene. I was leaving work and on my way to one of my classes at U of L. I made a few calls for them to see what they could do and informed them that they could call the crisis department of the police department and request a wellness check. Still, it was her decision whether she wanted help or not. That same day, I ended up in the hospital.

I had gotten so worked up that it triggered my asthma. Unfortunately, I had left my inhaler at work, so I was really in trouble. When class was over, I wrestled with whether I should go back to work to get my inhaler or if I should just try to make it home to my nebulizer. It was after school hours, and so it would be difficult to get back into the building to get to my classroom. Therefore, I decided to take my chances of getting home. It became more difficult for me to breathe, but I thought if I could just make it home, I would be okay. I made it home, but when I went to use my nebulizer, I realized the mouthpiece for the tube was missing. I tried to use it anyhow and felt it still should have worked, but it did not. I tried about three or four times, and I could not breathe. I knew I was in trouble and that I needed help right away. It was the worst feeling ever. I called 911 and began packing a bag as I knew I would more than likely be admitted. It seemed as if it took the ambulance forever to reach me. When I explained to them all that had taken place, the EMS worker decided it was best not to give me another treatment since I had already tried several. I cannot remember why he made this choice, but I did not think it was the best choice. The closest hospital was at least fifteen minutes away, and we would have to travel through a very busy part of the city during a very busy time of day. Instead of giving me another treatment, he simply pumped oxygen into my airways, but it did not work at all. I literally felt I was going to die. When I was a senior in high school, one time I had an attack so bad I passed out. I figured this was my body's way of protecting itself. I was praying and hoping I would pass out now while riding in the ambulance, but I did not. When I got to the hospital, the staff was told that my at home treatments did not work. They decided to intubate my lungs. I asked if they could put me to sleep to do that, and they informed me that I would be awake. I began crying and screaming asking them to please try a treatment one more time. They could not understand why I was in so much distress because my oxygen levels did not appear to be very low. This infuriated me as no matter what the machine read, I knew I could not breathe. I truly thought I was going to die. Finally, they agreed to try a breathing treatment one more time, and fortunately, it began working.

Things started to settle down. I was able to text my brother Mark and tell him where I was. I cannot remember exactly, but I think this was when he worked extremely early in the mornings and needed to get to bed early. I did not want to bother him, but I felt he needed to be informed. When he got to the hospital, he seemed to be upset with me that I had not called him first. I am sure he did not intend to make me feel this way, but I was made to feel as if having the attack was my fault. The doctors discussed putting me in the ICU to monitor me. My eyes filled with tears as I tried to tell my brother about my near death experience, but I could tell he was really tired, and so I allowed him to leave. I felt extremely alone. I wanted my mother, but she was gone. I slept off and on for most of the night and woke up still in the ER. I ended up going to an ICU room for a few hours before moving to a regular room. They kept me for about three days. I did not tell many people what was going on with me. I did tell my cousin Kelli and she and my cousin Angie, who I call my aunt, came to visit me. Mark was very helpful as well. He brought me things that I needed from home, including my laptop so I could do lesson plans. It is a shame that as a teacher, you cannot even rest when you are sick because you are worried about your classroom. My niece and sister-in-law at the time also visited with me, and she came to take me home when I was released.

I did not receive any visits from Michael or Derek. They were more concerned about Shellie, and I was of no use to them now. I did speak with Derek while I was in the hospital. I tried to explain to him that Shellie did not want to live and that the best thing they could do was keep her comfortable. I knew this because of her actions and also because of things she would say. She stopped taking her medication. She would often say that she wanted to go be with Mama. When a person is already terminally ill and has lost their will to live, there is not much you can do but support them. Michael and Derek were unwilling to do that, so there was not much else for me to do. A few days before she passed, I took Auntie to see her. When we came into the room, Michael was sitting next to her. He left, however, once we arrived. It upset Auntie that he and I did not speak, but she made it seem as if it was my fault, and it was not. What did he have to be upset with me about? I was the one who had paid thousands of dollars to bury our older brother. I was the one who had paid hundreds of dollars for my mother's headstone. I was the one who stood with my mother when they left her at hospice. I was the one who had endured all of their drama and dysfunction as a child and even as an adult, but still maintained a relationship with them out of respect for my mother and yet, he was upset with me. Why? Because I did not jump anymore every time you called? Because I did not save Shellie? I had put up a fence, and I was done with it. I was simply taking Auntie to say her final goodbyes. I was trying to do the right thing. The night before she died, I was there with my nephew. I specifically asked him if he wanted to be involved with any of the funeral arrangements, and he said no, that he would allow Michael to handle it. I asked him if he wanted to stay the night and offered to stay with him if he did. He did not want to, and so we both left. The next morning when I woke up, I saw I had missed a few calls from Mark. When I returned his call, he informed me that Shellie had died, that he had been to the hospital, and that everything was all over. I was extremely upset. I am hearing impaired and wear hearing aids, but I do not sleep with them, so I did not hear the call. At the time, we lived about seven minutes apart, I had wished that he would have come to get me. When I found out that Dayron was not there, I became extremely upset. I was not sure if he had been contacted and opted not to go or if he was simply uninformed. When I called Dayron, he let me know he was aware that his mother had passed and that he had found out about it on Facebook; Michael had posted. He did not contact family or anything. He just made the post. I was mortified, but then again, I should not have been because this is how they were, and this is how they did things. They did not care about anyone else. I asked Dayron if he wanted to go to the hospital to see if his mother was still there to see her one final time, and he said yes. I picked him up and drove him there, but we were told she had already been picked up by the funeral home. I took him home and went to Mark's as neither of us went to work that day. The longer we sat with what had happened, I believe Mark became more upset. His reasoning

102

for not coming to get me when he received the call was because he was worried we would not know anything if at least one of us was not there. I understood. We had both resolved that we would allow Michael and Derek to plan everything and to just show up like they usually did. Still, it did not sit well with Mark, or I that they did not tell her son that his mother had died.

Shellie and Dayron had a tumultuous relationship. She was on and off drugs and in and out of jail most of his childhood. As a result, he was raised by my mother. When my mother died, he moved in with his mother. By this time, he was eighteen or nineteen years old. They would have many disagreements. She would try to parent him as if he was still a child, and it just did not go well for them. Still, that was his mother, and he loved her. While at Mark's I got a phone call from Dayron. He was very upset. He no longer wished for Michael to do everything, especially considering how he had mistreated him. He wanted to know what he could do. So, I made a call to my friend's sister in Fort Wayne, Indiana, who worked at a funeral home. She informed me of my nephew's rights being her only child and told me to contact the funeral home to inform them of the situation. I contacted the funeral home, and we were able to intervene immediately. Mark and I took Dayron to the funeral home to discuss possible options. Of course, they had let her life insurance lapse, but she did have Medicaid, and there were certain expenses they would cover. We made the decision to have her cremated and to have a memorial service for her. When we went back to make the final arrangements, Dayron informed us that he had contacted Michael and Derek. I was very upset by this and knew things would not go well. Why would he do that when they did not even take the time to tell him his mother had died and were not planning to do so either? Dayron said he was trying to do the right thing and what Mama, my mother, would have wanted him to do by inviting them. That meeting did not go well. They kept trying to plan a funeral but had no means to do so. Derek offered a hundred dollars, which was probably her money, and Michael did not offer anything. He was very standoffish, short, and rather nasty. Derek did help with the obituary and seemed that he was trying to be cordial, but Michael would eventually turn his ear just as he had done with Shellie. She had even told me one time that she allowed him to get into her head and to turn her against me. By this time, I did not really care because it was a weight lifted off of my shoulders no longer having to deal with them. I was upset that Dayron had involved them, but I was trying my best to get through it.

Dayron was allowed a final opportunity to see his mother before she was cremated. Michael, Derek, and Mark had already seen her and said their goodbyes at the hospital; Dayron nor I had not. I pleaded with Mark to go to the funeral home with me as I had a feeling that things would not go well. When we arrived at the funeral home, they were not there, just Dayron, Mark, and me and we waited around for my oldest nephew, Adrian. In the process of waiting for him, Michael and Derek showed up. The atmosphere transformed immediately when they appeared. This was typical with them. It felt like an evil spirit had shown up, and I wanted to leave. Michael went on and on about how when this was over that he did not want anyone to say anything to him. I am not sure who he intended that for because I had already distanced myself from him completely by this time. Someone whom I had once been close to was now my enemy. Michael and I had become close when Mark was incarcerated. After losing his girlfriend to a brain aneurysm my senior year in high school, he turned his life around. He stopped drinking and using drugs, started going to church, and married a good woman. He distanced himself from the others, but somehow, we became divided again; the Harvey's (them), versus the Beeler's (us). I guess it was always that way. Derek approached Mark, Dayron, and me and said he needed to talk to us. He said it very harshly, "I need to talk to you, you, and you." Looking back at it, Mark and I both said we should have told him to check his tone. Nonetheless, we stepped into the hallway to hear what he had to say. He started loud talking and saying how he did not like how I came in and took over everything with HIS sister. He put his finger in my face, and when I put my hand up to move his finger out of my face, that is when he swung at me. I cannot remember if he made contact or not. I just remember that Mark intervened immediately. I remember hearing Mark say, "That's a female," and he and Derek started fighting immediately. I did not try to break it up. I couldn't have if I tried anyway.

Honestly, I was glad it was finally happening. It had been long overdue. This was not just about us helping our nephew, this was about over forty years of hatred they had for us for even being born. They had always resented our mother leaving their father to be with our father and to lead a better life. I never understood why they had been so upset because from what I knew from my mother and others, their father was like a demon. He was a true hellraiser. He fought my mother and abused them. He was a thief and never lived an honest life. My mother married him simply because she had become pregnant, and that is what they did back in those days. Regardless of the circumstances, it was not Mark nor my fault. We did not ask to be here, but they made our childhood make us wish we had not been. They were horrible to us. We could never have friends over because they were always there. They did not work. They did not contribute, and they were grown adults. It made things extremely difficult for my mother, but they did not care. Instinctively, I jumped in the fight to defend Mark. It was almost as if we were little children again, and I had to help my brother who was protecting me. Derek was throwing punches at me as well. When Michael came out, although he later lied to the court that he was trying to break it up, he immediately came at me. Fortunately, I had on a big feather coat; so, none of their punches really connected. I was able to step back when Michael came at me and hit him first. This kept him off me long enough before Mark, Adrian, or Dayron, I am not sure who, intervened. I kept yelling for the funeral staff to call the police, but they were in such shock they did not know what to do. Michael and Derek eventually fled the scene, but I was able to call the police still. I was in total shock. Here I was a grown woman who had managed not to be involved in any domestic disputes. No man I had dated had ever put his hands on me, and here I was now having to defend myself against my two older brothers, men who were supposed to love and protect me. How could this be?

At the same time, my adrenaline was pumping. I was elated that we had finally fought back and won. They could no longer intimidate us. We would not allow it. I ended up having to file a temporary restraining order against both of them to keep them from trying to attend the memorial. The funeral home was going to charge us extra to provide police security, so we moved the location. The memorial ended up being extremely beautiful. My nephew was pleased and that was all that matters. His job at the time had a special program then to provide funding for special scenarios such as this case. They provided the money that was needed to have her urn buried and to receive a small headstone. He would have a place to visit and to place flowers, and I was satisfied. I believe I experienced acute stress disorder following all of this.

The next day, I was extremely paranoid. As they ran out, I remember hearing Derek shout that this was not over. I was more concerned for Mark than I was for myself. I did not want him to be somewhere where Derek was and be attacked or hurt. I knew Derek was not really a fighter, but he was a street person; so, I did not know what to really expect. I remember going to the store and panicking because I thought I saw Michael. I remember buying mace, a baseball bat, and looking online at the process for purchasing a gun. It was really bad but fortunately, it only lasted a day. I met up with my hair stylist at the time. I needed to talk to someone, and she was a true woman of God, so I trusted her. She comforted me and encouraged me. She did not judge or shame me. She assured me that this was necessary, and that God was with me. She was right. Imagine fighting two men both over six feet and not having any major injuries and never falling to the ground. God was surely with me giving me strength and protecting me. This all happened around Christmas break, fortunately, I was able to be off work and school for a few weeks.

I was hopeful I would find peace during that time before returning to work and school. But once I went back, the depression returned. I am not sure if it was because of all that had taken place or if it was because of Seasonal

Affective Disorder. I just know I was struggling big time. I was extremely fatigued. It was hard to do anything. I was fortunate to have the same two professors in the spring semester as I had in the fall semester. I let them know about losing my sister, and they would extend some compassion toward me. After about a few months, I began to feel better and started getting back to myself in the classroom both as a teacher and as a student.

The court ended up picking up the case with my older siblings, and they decided to bring charges against them. It would be another year before we finally made it to court. They were not held liable, but at least they knew that I was not the one. They were used to fighting each other and nothing ever happening. At least with me, they knew if they tried that with me that the law would become involved. The judge did not hesitate to say that as well, that if there was ever another dispute to inform the court. I have seen them a few times since then, and no words or anything have ever been exchanged. Hopefully it will stay like that. I think it bothered Mark more than it did me because I had already seen them for who they were and started putting boundaries in place. I was more relieved than anything. I would never have to deal with them ever again in my life, ever.

Like clockwork, when the springtime came, I got better. I started going to the gym. I started eating better. I started losing weight and feeling better about myself. I was even open to dating now, and two men seemed to express an interest. That summer, I started dating one of them. The other I realized already had a girlfriend. The one guy and I did not date very long; he was not looking for a serious relationship, and I was not looking to play games. I felt pretty good about myself. I went to summer school for most of the summer and did not have much time off. I was, however, able to take a trip before the new school year and the fall semester. Once school resumed, I was in my groove. This year, I decided to make a change in my study schedule. Rather than spending most of my weekend studying and working, I decided I would get up a few hours early each day to read, study, or work on or grade papers and things worked out pretty well for me. I was in my second year working toward my MSSW at U of L. In addition to taking classes, I was also serving in my practicum as well. I tried to be optimistic, but my practicum was very disappointing. Before enrolling in the program, I made sure to consider and ask if the program was conducive for a full-time working student. I was assured that it was, but I found otherwise. The assignment I received did not give me any good practical experience. I spent little time with clients interviewing/assessing them and hours upon hours writing assessments to share with my supervisor. My supervisor was not even local, so I had no immediate feedback. He lived in Texas, I believe. We met on Saturday mornings via Zoom, and he would pick apart my assessments. No matter how long and detailed they were, they did not seem to be enough. As I talked with other students, I realized that what he was asking me to do was not realistic. I would never have a twenty plus page assessment of a client. It felt like I was given busy work to do. I was hardly learning anything. I spoke to my university advisor who agreed I needed a new assignment, only the next assignment was not much work or help either. The program I worked with was a good program. It was to support single fathers. But the work that I did, a teenager could do. I would basically take attendance, set up refreshments, and clean up. I did not gain much from either practicum experience. I am not sure if this brought me down or if it was the winter blues again, but by January of 2019, my depression would return full force. Only this time, I would not come out of it for a very long time.

CHAPTER 9

I Fell Apart

In January of 2019, the depression became extremely severe. It was hard to get out of bed. I did not even have the strength to shower. When it came to going to work, I would lie in bed for as long as I could. I would brush my teeth, put on some deodorant, and find something to wear that I did not have to iron. Anyone who knows me knows I iron everything I wear, even when it does not need ironing sometimes. Some days, I would repeat the same pair of pants multiple times in a week. I had lost track of when I wore what. I did not wear make-up, and I was not getting haircuts. Work was so challenging. I was starting to fall behind in my grading as well as with my school work at U of L. I shared with my department chair at work that I was struggling. I felt it was obvious I was off. I was missing deadlines to administer and grade assessments. Lesson planning became extremely overwhelming for me. I was just going through the motions just to get through the day. Finally, I went to my principal and shared with her that I was struggling as well. My principal at the time was Kim Morales. She was a huge support to me. She told me to let her know if there was anything she or others could do to support me. I was ashamed, but I felt my leaders needed to know. They had not had the opportunity to work with me in prior years. They did not know what a great teacher I really was. All they knew was this mediocre Lichelle who did not go above and beyond as she had during other school years at different schools and, I was ashamed of that. I was ashamed of what I thought they thought of me. I was ashamed I was not able to pull it together to do my job effectively. I did not want my students to suffer. I went to visit my doctor, the same doctor who took me off of work in 2015, and once again, I was encouraged to take time off work. I had some money in savings and thought I could manage for a little while. So, I followed her advice, and I took time off. When I shared this with my brother Mark, I felt his disappointment. I had wanted to stop attending classes at U of L as well, but I had a dear professor, Lori Paris, who convinced me otherwise. It was both a good and a bad decision. It was good because it gave me something to do other than lie in bed. It also showed me that someone else had compassion for me and that someone else saw my potential. I had Professor Paris for two other classes. I loved her passion and her teaching style. I learned so much from her. She was an excellent example to me of what a good therapist looked like. She was who I aspired to be.

She persuaded me to take advantage of the disability services offered through the university which would allow me extra time when completing assignments and tests. This particular semester, I had her for both classes, so that made it much easier. She told me that if I needed more time for assignments to take it and that if I did not feel up to coming to class to let her know and she would work with me. Her strongest argument was the fact that even in my struggle, I had maintained A's in both classes. She said it would have been different if I was failing or beginning to fail, but I was not. And so, I stayed. The only two things I did was go to class two days a week and to my practicum a few days each week. Aside from those two things, I was in bed. I am sure my classmates saw the spunk I once had fade away. It was painful to fake a smile anymore. I began to put on weight as I was making poor food choices. I had long stopped going to the gym as well. I began isolating. It had become a routine for me to connect with a few of my sorority sisters in the morning on my way to work, Ursula, Dede, and Dany but I had stopped doing that. I was not up to talking with anyone. I am not sure if I did or not, but usually when I am depressed, I deactivate my Facebook account. That is always a red flag for me by the way. The reason continuing with school this particular semester rather than withdrawing was a bad idea for me was because I was denied long-term disability as a result. My psychiatrist at the time was sure I would get it and encouraged me to take more time off work. Although she was wrong about me getting the long-term disability, she was not wrong that I was not ready to return to work. I had tried different medications and randomly went to therapy, but I had not done any healing.

That summer, my brother Mark thought it would be a good idea if I moved. They were raising the rent where I lived, and I was unhappy with the fact that we had a pool that was never open. They could never seem to find a lifeguard. I was not really in a place to make decisions for myself, and so I did what my brother said, and I moved. He, along with my nephew Dayron and my ex-boyfriend Trico helped me. Trico and I had been high school sweethearts. We were boyfriend and girlfriend from the end of my junior year through the end of my first semester of my sophomore year at Ball State. Like most young men, at least the ones I had known, he had issues with infidelity. We were in a long-distance relationship, and we were both going in different directions at that time in our lives. I had grown accustomed to the young men at Ball State while he had begun doing street activities. We broke up and went many years without talking but we were always connected through my brother. Trico was one of Mark's closest friends. He was a groomsman at Mark's wedding, and every major death that we experienced; our paternal grandmother, our oldest brother, our mother, and our sister, Trico was there for him. We would keep in touch from time to time. I always knew I was the one that got away and that he never stopped loving me. When my mother died in 2014, we exchanged numbers. He would call me when I went back to Arizona. He would check up on me and make me laugh. We would be on the phone for hours. This was much different from when we were younger. He never liked to be on the phone. We were always together anyway; so, it did not matter. When I came home for spring break the following year, he took me to dinner. And when I moved back home, we reconnected. We would go out to dinner sometimes, and I allowed him to come over to my house a few times. We tried to rekindle a romantic relationship, but it just was not there, at least not for me but we maintained a strong friendship.

That spring and summer of 2019, he would come over every week, Wednesdays I believe, to watch a television show called The Chi. He introduced me to the show, and I loved it. He would bring his Fire stick, and I would cook. He loved tacos. I would make him tacos, and he would act as if I was the greatest person in the world. He was about the only person I saw during that time, aside from my brother, his wife at the time, and his in-laws. With Trico, I could be just as I was. I did not have to pretend, and I was not made to feel ashamed. We never talked about my problems. Just his presence made all the difference. I remember him one time telling me that I was one of the two strongest women he knew; his mother was his first. I tried to return the favor and be a help to him as well. I was able to get food assistance, and I would buy him food. When his grandfather became ill, I encouraged him to go to the hospital and went with him. That was only the second time I had ever seen him cry. The first time was when I had tried to break up with him one time when he was being unfaithful. He was guilty, but he really was upset and did not want to lose me. I stayed that time. We were young then. We had shared so many things. He knew so much about my family and the struggles I went through with them. He knew what I came from and saw where I had gone. He was proud of me, and I knew that.

When it came time to return to work in the fall of 2019, although I was not ready, I returned. I had depleted all of my savings and had no other choice. My brother supported me financially the last month or so of the summer. Like usual, I felt pretty strong once the school year started. I had taken the summer off at U of L and decided to return. I did not want to delay my graduation even further. However, the first day I went to class, I knew it was a mistake. I barely had the strength to return to work. How was I going to be able to take classes again, not to mention a practicum? I waited until that Saturday to withdraw from classes and realized that I was one day too late. I would be financially responsible for the courses I had registered to take. I went through an appeals process and explained my situation with depression and was forgiven the responsibility of having to pay for the semester even though I was not attending. And so, I focused only on work. I did not know when I would be able to return to U of L. I was in survival mode. At this time, I had changed therapists. I did not feel that the other therapist was effective with me. She was Black and a minister. We shared a lot in common, but after taking classes at U of L, I felt that there was more she should have been doing with me. I felt that all we did was what I like to call, Talk Therapy. We would talk about whatever was on my mind that day. We did not seem to have a plan, which I had learned was essential from Professor Paris. It was also becoming too expensive for me to go as often as I needed. My friend, Sheryl, had told me about counseling services at the local seminary. The only thing was their therapists were marriage and family therapy students at the seminary. I decided to give it a try and would randomly go from time to time.

Most of that school year was a blur to me. I remember being extremely overwhelmed. It was as if everything and everyone in my building had sped up but me, and I was not picking up on things as quickly as I should have been. It was during this time I developed a severe phobia with technology. I was extremely intimidated by it and had a hard time learning the new systems and programs my school and team were using. During this particular school year, we had two planning periods a day. One of the planning periods was to be our regular planning time, and the other would be for various meetings and team planning. We only met for the extra planning period a few days a week. So, many days, I had a couple of hours without any teaching. The school day ended at 2:30 pm, but I would be finished with teaching around 12:30 pm. Every single day, I would leave work to go to Chick-fil-a. I would be starving by then, I no longer made or ate breakfast, but that was not the primary reason why I would leave each day. I would leave to escape from the responsibility and from the knowledge that I was not doing a very good job. I struggled with everything dealing with lesson planning, grading, classroom management, team assignments, and anything else I was tasked to do.

The second semester of that school year, 2020, brought something I would not be prepared for, and it was not just Covid-19 and the Pandemic. I had begun missing days at work. Many of the times, I would go to work, and then I would get there and realize I could not do it. So, I would call the secretary and tell her that I needed a substitute. I felt as if an anxiety attack was coming on every morning, and I knew my day would only get worse as I had my more challenging students in the later periods of the day. On this day, I left work early. I stopped by McDonald's to grab some breakfast and by Walgreens to buy some Benadryl. I wanted to eat and go to sleep and nothing more. At this time, I was also working part-time at Cato Fashion. I had made the decision back when the school year started, and I felt better. I wanted to pay off my debt and save up some money. I was still paying off the credit card I used to pay for my oldest brother's funeral back in 2012 as well as the flights I caught traveling back and forth to be with my mother while living in Arizona. I would go to work at Cato when I did not go to work at the school. It was harder to call off as we did not have many employees there. I had woken up and saw a text from my friend Carmen asking me if I was okay. I did not know what she was talking about. I then began to see missed calls from Mark and from Trikesha, Trico's younger sister. I knew something was wrong.

A few months back, Mark and I had become concerned that something bad had happened to Trico. Several days had gone by, and neither one of us had heard from him. So, I called Trikesha. They finally located him. He had been home the whole time. He was not working, and his phone had been disconnected. Trikesha and his mother checked on him and brought him food. That winter, he began working again and seemed to be doing better. I had seen him over my brother's during my Christmas break. He had told me he wanted me to help him with something concerning work, and I told him I would. A few weeks before this day, I had texted to ask when he was coming by my apartment. I was trying to help him with whatever it was before the spring semester started and I would be back to work. He told me he would come soon, but soon never came. After seeing Carmen's text, I called Mark and learned that Trico had died. From what I understood, he had visited with a lady friend and left for home but never made it. He died in his car right in front of her home. This was a very painful death to experience, but it would not be the first. I had lost so many others in addition to my oldest brother, my sister, and my mother. In a few years' time, I had also lost my spiritual mother, Debra Byrd, my spiritual father, Daniel Byrd, Carmen's parents who were like my parents, Charlie Sr. and Joyce Swain, Carmen's uncle who was like my uncle,

Charles Dunbar, three aunts, Helen and Clara "Bonnie" Ramsey and Jennifer Biggers, and uncle Greg Kimbro, two cousins, Kirk Lawrence and Curt Lockhart, two sorority sisters, Yolanda Wright and Amber Jones-Chamber, and I am sure I am missing others. Trico would be one of three that I would lose in 2020. I would also lose my dear friend and college brother Richard Casey and Carmen's brother who was like my brother, Charlie "Chuckie" Swain, Jr. Trico's death at the beginning of 2020 was a foreshadowing of what my year would become.

When Covid-19 hit and schools shut down, initially, I was relieved. I was depressed. I had lost touch with what was going on in the world. I just knew I was exhausted and could use the break. The original plan was to be out for three weeks; one week for spring break and an additional two weeks. Only, we would be out for the remainder of the school year and would not return until the fall. I thought I would use some of the time to rest and regain my strength but that I would use the bulk of my time off to plan lessons for the remainder of the school year and to get back on track, but that did not happen. It was as if I got into bed and never got out. School became virtual. I did the absolute minimum. I attended the required meetings, with my camera off obviously. I made the weekly assignments, but I hardly did any grading. We were supposed to make parent contacts on a regular basis, which I did not do. If they would have known the work I was not doing, I would have been in serious trouble. I would try to get out of bed to do work. I would only be up for a half hour or an hour maybe before getting back into bed. I would sleep all day and be up all night. It became a vicious cycle. I was not showering. I was not cleaning my apartment. I was not doing anything. I isolated myself from everyone, which was not a major alarm, as we were in a Pandemic, and everyone was trying to figure things out. I gained even more weight. My eating habits were terrible. I would wait until it became dark to go to a fast food restaurant, such as Zaxby's, Burger King, McDonald's, or Subway. I would go to the gas station and buy tons of junk food potato chips, Little Debbie snack cakes, candy bars, and diet soda. I did this so often one of the workers knew me. She thought I worked the night shift, and I allowed her to believe that. My apartment was beyond despicable. I was not taking out the trash. I was not washing dishes. I was not washing clothes. I had an infestation of gnats. You would think that would have bothered me, but I was too tired to do anything about it. Mark would come by, and I would try to straighten my living room and bathroom areas. My bedroom was horrendous, and I would not allow him to see that at all. One time, however, when he offered to come help me clean, I allowed him. We took one room at a time. We set off bombs to kill the gnats and put up sticky strips to catch any remaining. He encouraged me to get out and walk, and I would try to for a little bit. I would walk around my apartment complex, and I would be so tired I would not even shower. And I wore the same pair of pants and T-shirts every day. The only time I would shower and change clothes would be whenever Mark invited me over to watch a movie.

I am sure everyone saw the difference in me. Mark's mother-in-law and I would talk. She would remind me that if I needed someone to talk to that I could talk to her, and although I appreciated it, I never really took advantage of that opportunity. I was ashamed. I thought that being off that summer would allow me to regain my strength, but that did not happen. I only grew worse. And on August 10, 2020, when I was to report to return to work, I did not. I was a no call and a no show for three straight days. I was not even fully aware of when I was supposed to return to work as I had been avoiding my email like the plague. Finally, I checked and realized that I, in fact, should have returned to work. I texted Mark and told him that I was supposed to report back to work on Monday. It was Wednesday. He told me that he would be over that night and that the next day, I needed to call my job and go to the hospital. I did call my job, but I did not go to the hospital immediately. I contacted my psychiatrist and resumed taking my medication. I wanted to give myself a week to see if the medication made a difference, but it did not. I only had about eleven sick days, and those were about to end. I can honestly say now that I did not go to the hospital to get help as much as I went to save my job. It would be the third time in six school years that I had to use FMLA.

This was serious. My hospital stay was not very much help. They did not do much more than what my psychiatrist was already doing. We did not have much activity. The therapy that we did was in groups, and the things they were discussing I had already learned through previous therapy experiences. I listened to others share. Most shared about their experience with drug addiction or domestic abuse. In fact, this time, I really did not know what had brought on the depression. For the past several years, I experienced more down than up. From August through about November, I would be okay. Then from November through about April, I would be down again. I would muster up enough strength to finish out the school year in May, but I would struggle again in the summer until school resumed in August. I repeated this cycle for many years.

I backtracked to understand when this episode began. I determined that it had come on toward the end of 2018. I was very confused by it because nothing was wrong in my life at this time; everything seemed to be going well. I was doing well as a teacher and as a student. I was exercising, dieting, and losing weight. I had some experience with dating and was more open to it, something I had not been in forever. Things were really going well, but in spite of that, my depression still returned, and I was angry about it. My psychiatrist was beginning to think that my depression was resistant to medication. It would seem to work for a little while, but then it would stop working, or I would experience some major side effect and have to start all over again. I did not understand why this was happening to me. I remember saying to myself and to my therapist, what if I became unable to work and take care of myself? What would become of me then? It happened to my father, and he had three children to live for; so, what was going to keep it from happening to me. I had no children or husband, and I felt I had nothing and no one to live for anymore now that my mother was gone. I began to have suicidal thoughts. I did not want to kill myself or anything, but I wanted to die. I would wish that when I went to sleep that I just would not wake up. I wanted the pain to end. I was in so much pain.

At the same time that my world was falling apart, my brother Mark was going through things in his personal life as well. His marriage had ended. He decided to stay with me for a few months. This would give him time to find a new home, and he hoped it would make me feel better and take back control in my life. He found a new home, but I was not any better. He worked second shift; so, it was easy for me to pretend I was doing more than I was. He would not get home until about 11 pm. A few hours before then, I would get up, straighten up, and fix something to eat. I would be up when he came home, and I would stay up with him and watch television until he was ready to go to bed. I would sleep in until he was ready to get up. I would get up with him, but as soon as he left, I would get back in the bed. I wanted to do more, but I just could not. This time, I had more money saved up, and so I was not too worried about my finances. I was more worried about my future. What would I do if I could not go back to my job? Teaching is what I was trained to do, and it was all I had done professionally. I would think about other jobs I could pursue, without having to go back to school, but I was never able to figure anything out. I still wanted to be a therapist, but I was very unhappy about my practicum experience at U of L. And, although I had earned all A's in the twelve classes I had taken, I had not learned a whole lot, at least not about counseling. I did not like social work, and even though I knew I would be throwing two years of schooling away, I had no desire to finish that degree. When my brother found a house, he decided I would move with him. This way, I would not go through all of my money so quickly again. I had been saving to buy a home and was about to begin the process when the Pandemic hit. It was a good thing I did not because I would have purchased a home in Louisville based on Mark living there. Now that he was divorced, he decided to move back to Indiana, and I wanted to as well. The friends I did have lived in Indiana. I needed to build some sort of support system and social life outside of my sorority sisters and friends who all lived elsewhere.

Packing up and moving everything was a tall task. Mark became frustrated with me a few times when it did not appear that I was packing as quickly as I should have been. He had every right to feel that way, and I needed the push. It just maybe did not come out in a compassionate way, but he was doing the best he could. I did not want to be a burden on him, but that is exactly what I felt like I was becoming. I was so ashamed. Yet, I did not know what to do. I did not know where to begin. By this time, I was doing therapy virtually and was attending regularly, each week. Andrea was my student therapist at the time, and even though she was not licensed, she did the best she could, and she helped me. She kept me alive, literally. We would have sessions while Mark was at work so I could be open and honest about what I was feeling. As time went on, she realized I needed a higher level of care. She was also going to be graduating at the end of the semester, so she wanted to make sure she did not leave me without support. She stuck with me though. When I moved with Mark, most of my things remained in his garage. He set up my bedroom and a den area in one of his extra bedrooms. I did not unpack anything. I am sure he grew tired of that because one Saturday, he stacked all the boxes up in the back of the garage. It made it difficult for me to get to things, but I know he was only trying to be organized, and if I had not accessed those things by now, I probably was not going to for some time. I know he was extremely frustrated with me. Here he was going through a divorce and having to start over, and here I was a burden living with him without any plan whatsoever.

He did not know I did not care about life anymore, and I could not tell him that. He attended a therapy session with me and Andrea once, but I am not sure how much insight that gave him. I am sure he did not know what to do to help me. I did not even know what I needed. I did not really talk to anyone. Only my friend Michele even knew what was really going on with me, especially that I was not working and that I was now living with my brother. I felt like a visitor in Mark's home. He had redone the flooring and walls and everything and purchased new appliances and furniture. I did not want to mess things up or be in the way. I would talk to Michele from time to time. Prior to moving in with Mark, she would drive from Lexington to see me. The last time I saw her, I could see the concern, fear even, in her eyes. Even she did not know what to do. She was a part of a ministry called, The Well, led by Pastor Nina Anderson, an anointed woman of God I had met while living in Fort Wayne, Indiana. She now lived in Virginia and had a ministry that met virtually. Michele had invited me to attend the ministry's retreat the year before, but I did not. I did not have the strength nor the desire to do anything outside of what I had to do. This year, however, when she would invite me, I would consider it. I realized that if I was going to get better that the first thing I had to do was rebuild my relationship with God. Even prior to the Pandemic I had stopped going to church, and I certainly was not reading my Bible or praying on my own. There was an opportunity to win a free registration to attend the retreat, which was held both in person and virtually. I participated in the virtual drawing and won. I knew it was God and was hopeful that through this retreat, I would receive the teaching and prayer and encouragement I needed to get back up again.

I decided to get a hotel room for the weekend so I could be free to listen to everything without ear plugs and feel free to express myself however I saw fit. I knew there would be tears and lots of them. I had gotten so far away from God, and yet I loved Him very much and wanted to be close to him so badly. That retreat was the beginning of my restoration. I remember one of the ministers who was teaching, giving a prophetic word that there was someone who had been angry with God and that they needed to release it to Him because He knew already anyhow. I am not sure if she was speaking to anyone else or not, but she was definitely speaking to me. I was angry with God, but I was too fearful to tell Him. Who was I to be mad at God, and for what? I was angry because my plans had not worked out. I wanted to go to seminary to become a Pastor, not go to Hollywood to become a famous actor. Every time I tried to get back up to continue on with my life after that, it was as if I would get knocked back down with all of the deaths that I experienced. I did not have time to get over one death before another would come. Why was this? After all, He was God and could make it so that things worked in my favor instead of against me. That weekend, I released what I had been holding captive for over ten years, and God began to show me my path to healing and restoration. I shared some of this with Mark, but not all. I knew he would not understand, as we did not agree when it came to matters of spirituality and church. He felt I needed to be doing more practical things to get myself together. He did not understand that without God, I could not get up, and so, slowly but surely, I stopped sharing my journey with him.

I had made it up in my mind I was going to get up, and I began taking steps, small steps, but steps nonetheless. I reached out to my friend Carmen about a weight loss product she was now selling. I began using the product and went on a 1200 calorie a day diet. In a month's time, I saw some progress, but not as much as I thought I should. I decided to talk to my doctor about vitamins I could take to help give me the energy I needed to exercise to speed things up. Things seemed to be looking up for me, but things were starting to grow worse between my brother and me. He was irritated with me, and I knew it. I could not help but to feel it. Things seemed to change drastically from how things were when he stayed with me. He began seeing a lady friend, and I really felt uncomfortable. By this time, I was at my heaviest weight. I did want anyone to see me. I would stay in my room when she would visit, and if I was out when she came over, I would try to stay out until she left. I felt even more in the way now. I did a few things that infuriated him. One time when I came home, he asked me to wait about twenty minutes and to turn the sprinkler off in his front lawn. He had just put some product down and was trying to restore his yard. It looked bad then, but it looks really good now. He studied a lot and learned what to do to regrow it, and he did it all by himself. I had a virtual therapy session and forgot to turn the water off. He called me because he saw on his phone through his cameras and security system that the water was still on and told me to turn it off. He was very angry and there was nothing I could do about it. I offered to pay the water bill, but nothing I offered seemed to help. I understood his frustration, but I do not think he understood me at this time. He saw the outside, but he could not see my brain. It was so messed up. He was asking me to do something that would have otherwise been extremely simple, but it was not. I was no longer the responsible person I once was. I knew he wanted me to be, but I was not, and no amount of frustration could make me be. I knew he was also frustrated with me because of how loud my television would be. I would try to keep it low, but it was not low enough. I eventually purchased earplugs and would listen to my laptop sometimes. Otherwise, I would not listen to anything out of fear that it would disturb him. I could not tell what was too loud. The final straw was one day when I was putting away my groceries and one of the cabinets came off the hinges. He had painted and restored the cabinets himself and put a lot of work into them. I knew he would be heated. I knew I had to tell him but did not know when or how. I did not want to call and disturb him at work. I did not want to bother him as soon as he came home. I was going to wait until the next day, but he saw it that night before I had a chance to say anything. I think in his mind he had told me not to use that cabinet, but he had not. I was trying to use only one side of the cabinet with my food. I had never used this particular cabinet before. I did not break it. It literally came off the hinge as soon as I opened the door, but I knew he would not see it this way. He came to my room with a look of disgust. I had been seeing this often. He had this same look one morning when I had a migraine and had texted to ask him to bring me a cup of coffee and some Tylenol, something he had taught me. It was bad. When I reached for the cup, some of the coffee spilled in my bed. He sighed and shook his head in frustration. I could not do anything right, is what I thought. When I got up to explain the situation with the cabinet, it was as if he did not hear anything I said. I did not feel like an adult who was explaining to another sensible adult an unintentional accident that had occurred. I felt like a little child who had broken her older brother's toy, and I was in big trouble. I do not remember everything as he scolded me, but the one thing I do remember him saying was that he would never have anything nice (with me around). He went into his room and slammed his door. This crushed my very soul. How would I recover from this? I did not know how, and I did not know what to do. All I could think to do was leave, only I did not have anywhere to go. I called Michele and told her what had happened and decided to go to the hotel where I had stayed during the virtual retreat. I called my therapist as well. I had a new therapist now, and we were still getting acquainted with one another. It was at this very moment I realized that I had to get up, and sooner than I thought, not because I felt inspired to, but because I had no other choice. I did not really have anybody, not even Mark anymore. It hurt me to my core, but it would be the motivation I truly needed. I fell apart, but God would use that very same thing to put me back together again.

CHAPTER 10

I Got Up and Came Out of the Darkness

I stayed at the hotel for several days. I was so hurt. I did not want to face my brother. I felt defeated, and I felt as if I was at his mercy. After all, I was now living in his home, I did not have a job, and I had nowhere else to go. I thought about trying to get my own apartment. I did not have any income, but I was still employed, and I did have the money to do it. I would have to go back to work sooner than I thought, but it was better than having to stay there with the pain I was now experiencing. I figured my best option would be to try to go back to the apartments I had recently left in Louisville. I left in good standing, as I always strive to do. Surely, they would allow me to come back, and perhaps I would not have to go through the application process again for them to realize I did not have any income and technically could not afford to live there. When I called the apartments, the leasing manager remembered me right away. Unfortunately, someone had moved into my old apartment, and there were not any vacancies. People were staying put during the Pandemic. I would run into this problem several times trying to look for an apartment later as well. Again, the only people who knew where I was were Michele and my new therapist at the time. Both of them called to check on me. I did not have any answers, only tears and devastation. After several days, I realized I needed to go back to my brother's. I had probably spent five hundred dollars just in those few days, and I did not want to go through my money that quickly. The same day I was determined to go back, Mark texted me and told me we needed to talk and to come home. It did not feel like home to me, but it was the only home I had; so, I went back. I dreaded our conversation. He had a way of talking at me and not to me. He was my big brother, and what he thought or said far outweighed anything I thought or said. I was never good at confrontation or conflict with anyone, and this would not be any different. I tried to go over in my head what I would say, guessing what he would say and how I would respond. It was not anything I could really prepare for, however. I just knew that I would listen, but that I would also defend myself. I had made up my mind in that hotel room that I would have to heal now so that I could leave and not have to endure this type of pain ever again.

Mark shared his frustrations with me over the past few months; my television being too loud, me leaving the water running outside that one day, and me breaking the cabinet and not telling him until he approached me. I tried to explain to him why I waited to tell him, that it never seemed like a good time to talk to him about anything, especially not anything bad. He shared with me his disappointment with me leaving and not telling him for days where I was. He said he knew I was suicidal and how it was wrong for me to lead him to believe something could have possibly happened to me. I explained to him that someone knew where I was, that I was not just out there without any contact or accountability to anyone. I did not share this, but I remember thinking if he truly thought I was suicidal, he would not have treated me the way he did. He said he knew I was in a sensitive place and that he was trying to be careful with what he said to me. He said he had basically been holding his tongue on a lot of things. I do not remember everything he said. I do remember he talked a lot, and I listened. I tried to wait for my turn to speak. I also wanted to hear what was truly in his heart. I do not remember everything I said, but I did say a few key things. I apologized for the things I had done to upset him and shared that I had tried to rectify things. I had offered to pay the water bill and to pay to fix whatever damage the extra watering may have done to the yard. I had bought earphones and had actually stopped watching much television at this point and I offered to fix the cabinet. He said he did not want the money but that he basically wanted me to continue getting my life together, which I appreciated. I did tell him something he did not like. I told him he really did not know me, and it was true. He did not know me when I lived in Fort Wayne and was at my strength. He knew the broken me. He knew the struggling with depression me. He did not know me at all, but I told him I would show him who I really am and that I would never allow myself to ever be in this position again where I got so low, I had to depend on anyone. This was one of the reasons I had not wanted to move with him. We both had good intentions, but it went very bad rather quickly. I remember him calling what I had said to him "bullshit". I guess he saw it as me being arrogant, but that was not my intention. I was trying to explain that I would now fight with everything in me to get up out of the pit I was in and that this would be my motivation.

Things were uncomfortable for a long while, but God made me stay there for several more months before he would allow me to leave. I turned all the way up and little by little, I began to come out of the darkness and reclaim my life. I do not remember the order of things necessarily, but I became very serious about my spirituality and personal devotion to God. I became more committed to taking my medication and vitamins. I began exercising more consistently and rejoined Weight Watchers. And I started working toward a plan for me to regain income while remaining off work. Pastor Nina Anderson and The Well Ministry were a great support to me. I would wake up every morning to partake in Bible study and Praying the Psalms with Pastor Nina on Facebook Live. It was so refreshing to see some familiar faces. Hearing the Word of God and praying with the other women gave me life, and I needed it now more than ever. Michele became a true intercessor for me. I shared my desires with her and bathed them in prayer. She had faith for God to move in my situation, which made me believe too. Even though I had been denied before, I applied again to receive long-term disability. It was a benefit offered through my job. It would require communication with me as well as with my psychiatrist and therapist who were supportive of me. This is, I believe when I developed the theme, I carried for the remainder of 2021. I began praying and speaking Daniel Chapter 3, that I knew God was able and that He would move on my behalf, but that even if He did not, I was not going to bow down. I was not going to lose my praise, not this time. It had happened before where God did not answer my prayer in the way in which I thought He should, and I became extremely depressed. I was not going to allow myself to do that anymore. I was going to yet praise Him and trust He had a better plan for me. And so, I continued to face each day believing that God was behind the scenes working things out for me.

I started spending as much time as I could away from home. My brother worked the second shift. Initially, he would wake up between 11:00 and Noon, but he had started getting up earlier while he was trying to revitalize his yard. So, I would leave as soon as the sun came up. Primarily, I spent a lot of time at the public library in Clarksville. It had been my safe haven when I had broken my ankle years ago. Plus, it was near where my mother had lived before she became ill and moved with my sister. At the library, I was able to reserve a meeting or study room for several hours. With the time spent there, I would do my therapy sessions virtually, I would look for an apartment, I would read my Bible and other books, I would pray, and I would conduct whatever other business I could. One day, I came across an advertisement for the American Cancer Society. It was a virtual walk-a thon to raise money for cancer research. The goal was to walk forty miles the month of May and to raise a minimum of two hundred dollars. I had no idea that this would be the catalyst for my weight loss journey when I signed up, but it became just that. I made a commitment to walk a minimum of 1.3 miles per day. I would mainly walk at an outdoor park in Clarksville. It was close to the library and to where my mother had lived. I felt safe there. I used the time as an opportunity to pray for cancer patients, for those in healthcare providing care for cancer patients, for research, for caretakers, and for those who had lost loved ones to cancer. I reached out to my Facebook followers to encourage others to donate to the cause and to share names of those who needed prayer. It may not seem like much, but it was a big undertaking for me. It was important for me not only to begin this challenge but to finish it; for I had not been able to finish anything I started in a long while.

During this time, a lot of other huge things happened to me and for me. The day finally came when I was to receive the answer to whether or not I would receive the long-term disability. I had been in prayer that morning and worshiping God. I told him how I trusted Him, and I asked him to prepare my heart to yet love Him even if the answer was no.

Only, the answer would be yes. I was so overwhelmed with joy. I called Michele and shared the good news with her immediately. I had now been without income for nearly eight months, and my savings were beginning to be depleted. Fortunately, because I was living with my brother, I did not have any major expenses. He did not ask that I commit to any of the household bills. I just paid for my own expenses, including my car insurance, my cell phone, the hospital bill I had acquired, and food and other necessities. That was a tremendous blessing to me and allowed me not to spend my money too quickly. Not only was I being given a monthly income, I would also receive back pay going all the way back to September of 2020 when I last received a paycheck. My income would only be a portion of what I was making when I was working, I believe 66.7%, but it was a big increase from no income. Now, I could look for a place to stay.

It would be another five months, however, before God would allow me to move. I believe He made me stay right there to heal where I was. I had become a runner. I ran from Fort Wayne when things got tough. I ran from home to Arizona. I ran from Arizona back home and, I was trying to run now, but God would not allow it. He made me stay and work on my healing right there at the place where I had been hurt. Being awarded the money increased my faith and made me believe God truly was with me and that He was giving me the time I needed to truly heal this time.

A few weeks later, while driving home after getting a haircut, I was in a bad accident that left my car totaled. I had my car for close to ten years. It was paid off, and it had no major troubles. Once again, I was left with nothing but to trust God. I would not go to my brother to help me find a car. We had hardly been speaking. I would leave the house before he woke up and would be in bed when he got home from work. I would even do this on the weekends. When I did see him, I would be respectful and speak. I could feel the animosity between us. He probably thought I was being very disrespectful in his house, but I was trying to stay out of the way and trying to remain in a good head space. I did not have time to deal with what was going on between us. I had a bigger battle to fight, the fight for my life.

It took me exactly one week, but I found a car. I prayed and asked God for wisdom and for patience. I went to a few dealers. I finally met a young man that Sheryl had told me about. I called Alvin, Michele's husband, and he gave me some helpful advice as to what to look for, what I should put down, and my payment agreement. Even though I would only be given a rental from the insurance company only for so long, I would not be impulsive or desperate as I had been in the past when searching for a car. This time, I would pick what I wanted and not just take what I could get. My credit was good, and I had the money to make a good down payment, enough to lower my payments to a very low price. I could have paid for the truck in cash, but with me still working on my healing and not knowing when I would go back to work, I did not want to go through all of my money, so I put down what I felt was sufficient, and I was approved. I immediately took my car to my church's parking lot where I dedicated it to the Lord and prayed a prayer I had found online. I prayed that it would be a blessing and not a curse to me. I prayed that I would be able to make the payments. I prayed that it would be a reminder to me of the goodness of God. I had no plans on getting a new car, but I was very pleased with what I had gotten. It was an SUV, something I had been wanting for a long time, and it looked really good. I would later see how God does truly cause the bad things that happen to us to work together for our good when we love Him and are called according to His purpose.

Eight months later, when my father would be diagnosed with cancer and I would become his Power of Attorney, I would use my truck to transport him and his wheelchair to numerous appointments. His wheelchair would have never fit into my Elantra's trunk. This was the blessing I had prayed for my new truck to be, and I was grateful. I made a Facebook post thanking those who had been instrumental in getting my truck. I thanked the salesman, Michele Alvin, and even though he was not involved in the process at all, I did not ask him, and he did not offer, I thanked Mark. Through watching him over time and in various situations, I learned to research things and to exercise patience. I aimed to apply those skills when searching for my truck, and they served me well.

Things continued to go well for me. I finished the walk-a-thon challenge and well over the minimum requirement. I was feeling better, and I was doing much better. I was confident in the things I had put into place to ensure my continued healing my participation in the Well Ministry, taking my medication and vitamins, improving my eating habits and consistent exercise. I even began using mood light therapy which helped me tremendously. This is a lamp you can purchase to help give you similar light that we receive from the sun. I felt the difference. I had an energy I had not had in years, and I was hopeful again for my future. My doctor and therapist agreed I was not yet ready to return to work, and so I continued to receive long-term disability, and what a blessing it was. The longest I could receive those benefits would be two years. I had already received payments for the first year, and I would take advantage of the opportunity for a second year as well.

I began looking for an apartment, but it was a slow process. People were not moving around a whole lot due to the Pandemic. Apartments were also using a new tactic I had not experienced before when apartment hunting. They would have applicants pay a security deposit just to view an apartment, which was non-refundable. I learned this by not reading the small print for an apartment I did not want after seeing it. I was disappointed, but I did not get angry. I just asked the Lord for greater wisdom and patience and for Him to restore the four hundred dollars I had lost.

That summer, I would experience two additional family deaths. Two of my cousins that were near and dear to my heart would die from Covid-19 complications. It was devastating to our family, both of them were only children and had only reached the age of fifty years old. What made it even more devastating was that they were such good people. They loved the Lord, and they loved their family. Aaron "Rusty" and Monica's deaths did something to me I had never experienced before. I completely lost my appetite. I remember going to the doctor during this time and him doing labs. Those labs showed I was suffering from malnutrition. I was completely blown away. How was it possible for me to experience this when I was overweight? Well, it was possible, and that possibility became my reality.

For weeks, I lived off pudding and applesauce and protein shakes. It was all I could do to have some sort of nourishment and to keep my cousin Kelli from fussing me out. I lost almost twelve pounds in two weeks. This happened right before my friend Mary's wedding. I had literally just bought a dress and tried it on about a week before the wedding. When I put it on, on her wedding day, however, it swallowed me. Others thought this was a great thing. After all, I was overweight, and I had been working to lose weight, but I knew this was unhealthy and that I had to do something about it. I was not even exercising anymore and was losing this weight. I had to start eating again, and slowly, but surely, I did. I got really sick right before the wedding. I thought I was having an asthma flare, and Mark drove me to the ER. I was diagnosed with pneumonia but was said to have not been contagious. I was prescribed antibiotics and steroids. I took the medication and got better, but as usual, I also gained some weight. I would get it off in a few weeks though. Looking back at it, I felt I did not have pneumonia but that I had Covid-19. I say this for a few reasons. When I went to visit a pulmonologist and he reviewed my X-rays, he agreed that it had not been pneumonia. My primary care doctor said it was probably the virus but that it was undetected. I had been vaccinated, but I knew it was still possible to get the virus. I also later did have the virus the following winter, and it felt very similar to that. Nevertheless, I made it through the wedding and through my family deaths and continued on my journey. I would become more involved with my cousin Emma. I call her aunt, but she is actually my mother's first cousin. Aaron "Rusty" was her son. She did not have any other children, and her husband had died years ago. All she had was our family, and I would do my best to be there for her. I still do my best to this day. I continued to be consistent with my goals and continued to remain hopeful that God would lead me to an apartment where I would be satisfied.

I finally found a place in October. By this time, I was sharing little information with my brother. I had just told him that I was looking for an apartment and that I had the means to pay for it. Things were getting a little better between us. When I bought my car in May, I received a smoker as a free gift. I thought about giving it to Alvin as a gift for the encouragement he had given me, but I decided to give it to Mark. It was his birthday and what better gesture than to give him something as a blessing to his new home. I presented the smoker to him as well as some cupcakes, and he was pleased. This was my genuine effort in trying to do my part to be at peace and to heal both our relationship and myself. That, as well as my cousins' deaths, opened up the door for us to begin talking more. I realized I was not the only person going through something. He had gone through a divorce and had given up everything he had worked for, including his home. He had to go through the process of buying another home and he did all of this while trying to look out for his little sister who was battling depression. I knew he loved me and that he did not intend to hurt me. Yet, that did not erase the hurt I experienced nor the distance I was feeling now, distance I created in order to protect myself from any further pain. When I finally found my apartment, I pledged I would not ask for any help. The only thing I would need him to do would be to help clear out a way in the garage for my things to be moved. I had purchased a new living room and bedroom set and had plans to give my furniture to my nephew Dayron. I boxed up everything and paid movers to move all my things. All they had to move were about twenty boxes plus my mattress and box spring and my washer and dryer. I paid more than I probably should have, but at this point, I did not have any other option. I cleaned my bedroom, the bathroom I used, and the other bedroom I used as a den thoroughly. I paid to have the carpet cleaned. I helped move my furniture that was for Dayron into the garage so that he would not have to come into his house. Dayron moving his things was delayed a little bit because he had contracted the Virus, and we wanted to be safe.

A few days before moving day, I felt some heaviness trying to set it. I think I was overwhelmed with the packing had to do. I had started losing weight, and so I had more clothes than when I first moved with my brother. Plus, I had toiletries and other things I had been using. I do believe I laid in bed for a day or two. My friend Natasha would eventually encourage me to get up, and she helped hold me accountable to getting things done. The last thing I did for myself, prior to me leaving, was to develop a wellness/crisis plan. I had learned about this when I did training to receive my peer support specialist certification a few weeks prior. In the plan, it indicated how things were when I was well, how things were when I was not well, and things that would help me to become well again. I shared a copy with Mark as well as with a few other people, including my doctor, my therapist, and my friends Michele, Natasha, and my Kelli. I would be living by myself again. No extra set of eyes would be on me anymore to see when I was down. All they had to go by was what I shared with them, and I had to commit to doing so honestly and completely. Moving into my new apartment gave me an excitement I had been missing. I had been longing for my own space. I never intended to stay with my brother for as long as I did. I was now in my own space and could create my own routines and way of living that would benefit me. I did not have a dining room set initially. The one I had originally picked out, I put back because it was not what I really wanted. I was done with buying things for the sake of having something. And so, I waited. This actually turned out to be a good thing because I was able to use the dining area to store all of my boxes, and in a few days, I would have emptied every box. I was able to separate my clothes by season and try them on to see what I could still wear or potentially still wear. I bagged a lot of clothes and shoes, and for the first time ever, I donated those clothes and shoes. In past years, I literally just threw things away just to get them out of my sight, but I had time now, and I took full advantage of it. I organized my closet, and I was so proud of it. It was the best looking closet I had ever had. I was fortunate to have a storage room on my back patio. I hung my fall/winter clothes in my closet and placed them in my drawers and stored my spring/summer clothes in my storage closet. It felt so good to have everything organized and clean.

For the first time in years, I would have a good winter season.

I celebrated the holidays with my cousin Kelli, Emma, Angie, and others. I had spent many holidays with Mark's former in-laws, and not that it was bad to be with them, but it felt so good to be with my own family again. I decided I wanted to celebrate Christmas Eve with my immediate family. I invited my father, my brother Mark, my nieces and nephews, and their children. Not everyone came, but it was still a beautiful day. I made breakfast, and I gave gifts to my father, my brother, my nephew, and my great-niece and great-nephews. I made it a point to really celebrate Mark. When I moved, I offered to buy him a washer and dryer, because we had been using mine, but he told me it was not necessary. The week after I had moved into my apartment, I invited him and his lady friend over. I served appetizers, and I gave him a gift. It was a massager to use for his legs and feet. He was a welder and worked hard. I thought this would help, and he said it did. For Christmas, I went all out. I bought him several things. I bought him a pair of nice shoes, a gift card to Macy's, a gift card for a massage, a set of U of L insulated cups, and tickets to a Lakers game in Atlanta against the Hawks. I would attend the game with him in January, and we had a blast. It was my way of saying thank you, I love you, and that I was not going to allow what had happened between us to change how I felt about him or how

I treated him. He was overwhelmed, and my mission was accomplished.

I was in a very good space and ready to bring in the New Year. 2021 had been the year of Surrender, but 2022 would be the year of Productivity. I was working with a new therapist now and developing that connection, and I had hired a life coach. Together, she was helping me to develop a mission and vision statement as well as some goals and an action plan. I was more determined now than ever. I had been working so hard to prove to my brother and others that I could get back up, and now I would work to prove to myself that I could remain standing up. 2021 started out being one of the worst years of my life, but I later realized that what I thought was the worst day of my life turned out to be the best day of my life because I got up, and I came out. Out of the darkness, and I intended to never go back there again.

CHAPTER 11

Where Do I Go From Here

2022 came in swinging! On January 1, 2022, I woke up full of hope to a phone call I thought was my daddy, but it was not. It was one of the staff members where he lived. They were calling to tell me that he had been falling and also experiencing rectal bleeding. I had to drive to Carrollton, Kentucky, which was about an hour to meet him at the hospital. He was admitted into the hospital. The cause of him falling was because he was suffering from anemia from losing blood, but they wanted to determine what was causing the bleeding. They wanted to perform a colonoscopy and an MRI. Initially, he opposed the colonoscopy when they presented it to him. But, once I arrived and was able to better explain things to him, essentially that he would be put to sleep for the procedure, he agreed. I was concerned about the bleeding because that was how things had started out with my mother's cancer, only her bleeding was vaginal from endometrial cancer. They were not able to do a full scope and biopsy because his bowels had not completely emptied from the medication provided before the procedure, but from what they did see, it was obvious he had some sort of tumor. Based on the surgeon's report, the tumor was extremely large and it was in a very awkward location, not in his colon but directly in his rectum. The doctor was pretty sure it was cancer. According to that surgeon, it would possibly be impossible to remove the tumor, and if so, Daddy would definitely need to wear a colostomy bag for the duration of his life. He would need to be able to have a complete colonoscopy before a diagnosis could even be made, which I was very concerned about. I learned that the place where he was living was not a skilled nursing facility. They simply provided shelter, food, and made sure residents were given their medication and were transported to their appointments, but they did not have registered nurses to ensure he took the colonoscopy prep medication and received the treatment he would now possibly need. It was decided he would go to a nursing facility rather than back to the group home where h he lived, possibly indefinitely. It would take a lot of work to finally get him the testing he needed to make the diagnosis, and it was strenuous. I worked with my brothers, but I was doing much of the leg work. When he first went to the new nursing facility in Carrollton, he supposedly tested positive for Covid-19 and had to be isolated for ten days. I was told he would still receive physical therapy while isolated. I was concerned because he had been in the hospital for several days, and I remembered how my mother was after a longer stay in the hospital. However, he did not receive any physical therapy. By the end of the ten days, that father who walked in the front door and who was using the restroom on his own was now in a wheelchair and wearing Depends. I was devastated. If he did have cancer, I did not want to see him go down that fast. I became his Power of Attorney and worked with Medicaid to ensure that his housing expenses would be covered. His medical care was already covered by the VA. For months, I drove up and down the highway to Carrollton, Kentucky, to see about my daddy. I put more miles on my new truck than I wanted to, but it was necessary, and I was thankful that I was able. Things moved very slowly in the beginning, and it took a long while to work through the systems, but we were finally able to have the complete colonoscopy and biopsy in March, and from that, we learned that it was in fact cancer. From the MRI, we also learned it was possibly Stage 2, but more than likely Stage 3, and he would need treatment as well as surgery. The surgeon in Carrollton was very honest with Mark and me that he was a general surgeon and that he did not specialize in oncology. We opted for a higher level of care, and he supported us. I began transporting him to Louisville to the VA. On days that he had appointments, I would be on the road for about four hours. It took one hour to get him, an hour to take him to his appointment, an hour to take him back to the nursing facility, and an hour to get back home. It was a lot. I tried very hard to maintain my strength. I had set some goals at the start of the year to put some things in place to help me not only in this situation but with my day to day. I committed to doing a daily devotion in which I would spend time studying the

Word of God and in prayer. That, in addition to the other habits I maintained from the previous year, such taking my medication and vitamins, eating right, exercising, communicating with my doctor, and going to therapy helped tremendously. Still, it was a lot to manage.

It seemed like it took forever for my father's Medicaid to be approved. They would ask for a certain document, and I would submit it, only for them to turn around and request something else. At the nursing home, they were misplacing his clothes, and so I was replacing them just as fast as they were misplacing them. My brothers Mark and Bryan gave their financial support as well. Bryan was my father's oldest son. He was not raised by my father and did not share the same close relationship Mark and I did, yet I still tried to respect him as the oldest and to keep him informed. In the beginning of everything, I sent frequent detailed messages to keep them up to date. We even had one or two conference calls via Zoom. I shared with them what was going on with him and what I was doing to support the care he needed. Having had to bear the responsibility of ensuring my mother's care and her final arrangements, I wanted to get ahead of everything. I contacted the funeral home to learn that process, and I also contacted the hospice where my mother was cared for to see if he was eligible for their services. Bryan felt that I was moving a little too fast, and maybe I was, but I knew that I would be the person shouldering most of the responsibility when my father died, whenever that was. And so, I was trying to do as much as I could now while I had my strength. I think Mark and I understood the situation a little more and a little sooner than Bryan had. We had been through this with our mother. Bryan was very hopeful that it was not cancer; even though I was sharing with him my conversations with the different doctors. When the results came back, I was not as shocked. I had already prepared myself. I was more surprised and relieved that a plan could be put into place and that his condition was not terminal. I met with three different oncologists, the oncologist in charge of his chemotherapy at the VA, the radiation oncologist at the U of L Brown Cancer Center, and the oncology surgeon at U of L Physicians. I transported my father to all those different consultations from Carrollton to Louisville, all except for one. One time I trusted the VA transportation to get him there, and I would meet them. However, they ended up taking him to the wrong appointment. I was in tears and so upset that the doctor agreed to meet with me since I was his POA, and it was just a consultation.

We did not begin treatment until April. The plan would be for him to receive about six chemotherapy treatments, then radiation, and then surgery. We were told it was possible he would need more treatment before the surgery. We were also told there would be a two month break in between him receiving radiation and the actual surgery. We were told he would need a colostomy bag after the surgery but that it would hopefully only be temporary. It was a lot of information to digest, and I had to do so alone most of the time. Mark worked second shift. He had also bought a new truck and was not sure if Daddy had the ability or strength to climb into it. So, I did the transporting. I also visited him to make sure he sometimes ate things that he liked he loves KFC, McDonalds, and pizza but to also ensure that the nursing staff were aware that he had someone who cared about him and that they needed to make sure they did the same. In May, I was finally able to relocate him to a nursing facility in Louisville, Kentucky. This would cut out a lot of my travel time as well as money I was spending in the cost of gas. I still would transport him to appointments for a long while because I did not trust others to get him where he needed to be on time. Once we learned that the nursing facility could now transport him, we started allowing them to transport him to the appointments that I could not make, and Mark would meet them there. I wanted to be certain that one of us was always there with him. He would not go through any of this alone. Where we stand now, he is about halfway through his radiation treatment. Once he is done with that, he will have two more chemo treatments, and then hopefully by Thanksgiving, he would have had his surgery. Of course, plans can change once they do more imaging if they find anything. The oncologist was confident that the cancer had not spread to any other organs or areas in his body, but after what I experienced with my mother, I know there is no way to really tell. All I can do is something my mother said to me years ago that I did not agree with initially but learned to accept, "hope for the best, but expect the worse".

For the most part, I have done pretty well through this road with my father for the past seven months. I believe it was because of the supports I already had in place that made the difference. In the past when tragedy struck, I was never really prepared and spent most of my time simply pushing through and surviving. Now, I had created some healthy habits and rather than just pushing through and surviving, I was thriving even in the face of a major obstacle. There have been a few days in which I have gotten down. I was concerned a few times when I found myself lying in the bed a little too long and getting away from my healthy habits, such as not doing my devotion and prayer, not taking my medication and vitamins, and not exercising. That is when I would reach out to my sisters, Michele and Natasha, and they would encourage me through it and help hold me accountable. One time, Michele came and visited me when I told her I was struggling. I guess she realized it was best to confront the situation immediately rather than to wait for things to build. The next time I told her I was struggling; I went to visit with her in Lexington. She offered to come to me again, but I wanted to save her a trip, and plus, I needed to get away for a bit. I would reach out to my friend Kelli when I wanted to get out of the house, and she would do things with me. We went to the comedy club, to a lounge, and to the cigar bars quite a few times. It was good now to let someone else into my life that was here locally and that I did not always have to drive out of town to Lexington, Fort Wayne, Chicago, or Atlanta just to get away for a spell.

Through this process, I learned that habits mean everything. When my spiritual mother, Debra Byrd died, I remember my spiritual father, Daniel Byrd, sharing how he maintained his daily devotion because that was something he had done for so long and that even during his pain, he continued. He taught about us having what he called our MDR, our Minimum Daily Requirement of the time we needed to spend with God and His Word in order to be alright. I was determined to find my MDR, and I would pursue it every day. As for my weight loss, I was not experiencing the success I had seen the year before. I had lost about sixty pounds in about eight months' time. But now, I was going up and down or at a standstill. This did disturb me, as I presently wanted to lose at least another fifty pounds. At the same time, I was not completely discouraged. I knew what I had been going through with my father, and I was proud that I at least had not gained an enormous amount of weight in the process as I had done in the past. In fact, from the time I returned home from Arizona in 2015 and the end of 2020, I had gained about eighty pounds. When I went to my current doctor, I was a whopping three hundred and eleven pounds. I could not believe it. I have lost about ten pounds this year for a total of about seventy pounds. I have a long way to go, but I have already come so far.

When I look back at the picture I took during my doctor visit in December of 2020, I can hardly believe what I see. It was not just the weight gain. There was no life in those eyes. I was truly the walking dead. My soul felt dead, like I was at the point of no return, and I did not know if I even wanted to make it back, but I did, and thank God for those who have stood with me. I am still working with my therapist regularly and maintaining my goals and the plans I put in place at the start of the year. I have accomplished so much. The fact that I am nearing the end of writing this book is a huge accomplishment. It was something I have wanted to do for a while. It took me a while, but once I began writing, it became easier for me. I had always been a good writer. My daddy had encouraged me to write when I was a child. I would write short stories all the time just so I would have something to share with him during our phone conversations. Sometimes, I would even write poetry. I think I wrote a short play once and two short novels. When I left to go to college, I left a box filled with all these stories I had written, mostly through elementary and middle school. And, when my mother moved out of my childhood home a few years after I graduated from college, the person helping her move mistakenly threw that box away. I did not realize it then, but subconsciously I lost my desire to write. I would write a poem here or there for my students or for special occasions, but I did not spend any real time with it anymore. Writing this book has been one of my greatest joys. It has allowed me to share my story with others in hopes of helping somebody. And, if I only help one person, I would have achieved my mission.

After much consideration and prayer, I decided I would not return to teaching this school year. At this time, I have now been on medical leave for the past two years, and I am not able to extend it any longer. I maintained my position for as long as I did partly because of the life insurance and the benefit of having a job so I could obtain an apartment, my new truck, and other necessities, but I also did it because I was not sure if I had the courage and strength to do what it was that I truly wanted to do. I wanted to go back to school, but not to finish the MSSW program. I wanted to pursue a Master of Art in marriage and family therapy at the local seminary. At U of L, I had completed two years of schooling and only needed one more year to finish, but it was not what I wanted to do. I was not passionate about it and it is very difficult for me to do anything in which I do not possess great passion. That would mean I would be starting over at the seminary to pursue a new degree. Perhaps one or two classes would transfer, but for the most part, I was starting over. I applied for the program and received a scholarship, and I will be starting school this fall. I will not be returning to the classroom. I will be resigning from my position and leaving the classroom hopefully forever.

Teaching has been my life. I did not actually realize what it had meant to me until I read Mrs. Viola Davis' book, Finding Me. In her book, she talked about her acting career and how it had been about more than just her acting but that it was about saving her life from the life that she knew and the obstacles that she had endured as a child. Teaching had been that for me. Becoming a teacher is what drove me through my childhood when things were tough. It was my motivation for getting good grades to go to college. It was my out and it served me well for many years. It was all I had ever done professionally since I was twenty-one years old. I had dreamed about it since I was a little girl. It was all I had known and yet, there was a new passion building on the inside of me, a new calling. I wanted to help other people who battled mental illness in the way I had. I had received a great deal of support, but I wanted to be an even greater support to others. My mission was now to share my story, to stand up for and with others, and to lend support in developing their inner peace, and becoming a licensed therapist would be my starting position. There is so much I want to do. Eventually, I want to have my own practice. I want to write more books. I want to tour the world, sharing my story and telling others how to come out of the darkness. One day, I would like to have a retreat center where people can go to heal from their depression. I want it to be a place where they would not have to worry about anything but their healing. It would be a place where they would learn some of the same healthy habits I learned and used to come out of my depression. I want to be the help that took me a very long time to receive. I try not to think about what I desire to do too much in order not to overwhelm myself.

I have been reading one book per month this year, and I am preparing to read a book entitled, Do It Afraid by Joyce Meyer. Fear can and has crippled me in so many ways. I get inside of my head and overthink things and see too much of the big picture without focusing on the small details and steps I simply need to take day by day to achieve my dreams. I know that I can do all things through Christ who gives me strength. As long as I have Him, I can face and overcome anything. My Pastor, Dr. Kevin Cosby, Sr., teaches that we can endure anything if we know it is not permanent. I totally believe that, and I add to that, we can also endure anything if we know we are not alone. Depression does not have to be permanent, and we do not have to battle it alone. That is the purpose in sharing my experiences, to let others know that I have lived through it, that I am now able to tell my story, and that with the right support and a lot of hard work, they can too.

Where do I go from here? Anywhere my heart desires. I have taken my power back, and I do not ever intend to lose it ever again. I will continue to fight for myself and for others, and together, we will have the victory.

CHAPTER 12

Conclusion

I wanted to use this final chapter to share how we can help others through their battle against depression. I am not an expert. I am not a licensed therapist, yet; nor have I done any major research at this time, but I do have experience as someone who has battled depression and as someone who has tried to help others. One of the first pieces of advice I would give is to understand that unless you are a doctor or a licensed therapist you are not an expert, and you should never try to present yourself as someone who completely knows and understands the impact of depression in one's life. The best thing we can do when trying to help others is to guide them toward seeking medical help. We can only be a support to them. We cannot give them the major tools they need and deserve. Many people struggle with the idea of taking medication for various reasons. I struggled for many years as well. I was a minister in the church and was made to feel like if I needed medication, it was because my faith was small and all I needed to do was seek God, stop sinning, and rebuke the enemy in my life, and I would be set free.

I tried other people's way for a long time, and it did not help me. I had to get to the place where it did not matter to me what others thought. I was sick and tired of being sick and tired, and I wanted it to end. Then, when I finally began taking medication, it took a long time to find the right medication for me. Some medications would not work at all. Some I would experience more negative side effects than any positive outcomes. Some would work for a short season, and then they would stop. I was extremely discouraged, which is why I kept starting and starting again. I did not realize what that was doing to my brain. Now, I tell everyone to never stop taking the medication abruptly or without being under a doctor's care. Last year, after trying different medications for nearly twelve years, I finally found something that worked. The problem with that, is that I experienced other side effects I had to consider. The medication caused my hair to thin, and it also caused my blood pressure to elevate. I had to make a decision of whether I was going to stop taking the medication that was helping me or if I was going to find a way to manage the side effects. My friend Sheryl, who is also a nurse, helped me to prioritize my mental health. The medication was working, and so I decided to stick with it. As a result, I would have to take a low dose blood pressure medication, and I would have to accept the fact that I would have to maintain a short hairstyle. My mental health has become the most important thing in my life next to my spirituality. In addition to finding the right medication, I also asked my doctor what specific vitamins I needed to take. I was told I needed B12, D3, and Folic Acid. So that is where

I would tell others to begin. I would tell them to see their doctor to learn what different medications and vitamins there are and what would best support them.

Keep in mind that we are not talking about people who are basically experiencing an episode of depression due to a particular situation, but we are talking about people who have experienced deep depression persistently and who have not been able to come out of it on their own. The thing we fail to understand about medication is that it does not fix our problems, but it restores a chemical balance in our brain so that we can think better to fix our own problems. Once I realized that, I had no trouble taking the medication and vitamins. Once a person's brain is working properly, he or she usually possesses the ability to do whatever else is required of them. They may need some support in sorting things out, and that is where a good therapist comes into play.

People always ask me how to find a good therapist, and I wish there was an easy answer, but there is not. I encourage people to either request a list of therapists from their insurance company or to go online to Psychology Today to review various therapists in their area. Talk to other people whom you may know that are in therapy and ask them to share their information. The current therapist I have now came as a result of me seeing an old high school classmate post about the practice which she received therapy on

Facebook. I asked for the information, and I made the call. You have to spend time with a therapist so they learn you and so that you can get a feel for whether or not it is a good connection, and this does not happen in one or two sessions. You have to be willing to be transparent and willing to walk through the process because it is a process. Your issues did not start overnight; therefore, they are not going to end that way either. Too many times we expect therapists to help us work through years of trauma, in just a few sessions and that is simply unrealistic and unfair. You will know it is a good connection because you will become more comfortable sharing with them.

I learned that part of having a good therapy session was for me to come prepared with topics I wanted to discuss, things that I wanted to work through, and goals that I wanted to accomplish. You cannot expect the therapist to do all of the work. We have to come up with an idea of what we want therapy to look like, and we have to be willing to do even more work in between our sessions. Ask for homework assignments, not just busy work, but assignments that will challenge you to think and to confront the way you process and approach certain situations. Therapy can work if you work it.

Let me add this for my Black sisters. You must eliminate the notion that you have to have a Black therapist in order for someone to be able to relate to your story. The purpose of therapy is not to make a new friend, and so you cannot approach it in that way. You simply want to work with someone who is skilled in working with people who are struggling with depression and who is effective in helping them overcome their challenges. Aside from your doctor or psychiatrist and your therapist, you want to develop a good support system. You cannot get through what you are going through alone, and you should not try to. You need to make sure you have more than one person you can rely on for support. Remember, they are there to support you, not to serve as your therapist Different people can offer different things to you. For example, my friends Michele and Natasha pray with me, they challenge my thinking, and they hold me accountable to my goals. Michele is a great support because she at one time served as a clinical social worker, and Natasha is a great support because she too has battled depression and anxiety. My friend Kelli gets me out of the house to do things, and if I called on her to help me do something, such as clean my apartment or see that I paid my bills, I know she would do just that. I have sorority sisters that check in with me on a regular basis through a phone app called Marco Polo. It allows me to leave and listen to messages at my own pace. It is a good tool for me. When I was working to obtain my Peer Support Specialist Certification, I learned about wellness and crisis plans. I liked them so much I decided to create one and to share them with those closest to me. The following is the wellness/crisis plan I created before I moved out into my own apartment.

WELLNESS

Lichelle L. Beeler

WELLNESS PLAN

For me, Recovery means I:
1. Am able to function independently on my own.
2. Am able to make healthy decisions.
3. Am working toward my goals.

Part 1: *Daily Maintenance Plan*
To stay well, every day I will:
1. Practice good hygiene.
2. Take my medication, including vitamins.
3. Use sun or light therapy.

To stay well, I may also…
1. Do some form of exercise.
2. Practice some form of spirituality, i.e. church, Bible study, prayer.
3. Socialize with others.

Part 2: *Planning for Triggers*

One of my most common triggers is:
1.   Death
To deal with this trigger, I will:
- Discuss in therapy + Daily Maintenance Plan

2.   Winter
To deal with this trigger, I will:
- Increase light therapy, increase vitamin intake, + Daily Maintenance Plan

3.   Fatigue
To deal with this trigger, I will:
- Consult psychiatrist/primary care + Daily Maintenance Plan

Part 3: *Early Warning Signs*
Three of my early warning signs most obvious to others are:
1.   Messy home, car, and workspace
2.   Poor hygiene
3.   Isolation

Three of my early warning signs hardest for others to notice are:
1.   Loss of interest /feelings of hopelessness
2.   Inability to make decisions

3.   Inability to pay bills and handle other necessary business

When someone points an early warning sign out to me, or I notice one myself, I will:

- Seek support from my therapist, psychiatrist/primary care, and other support systems.

Part 4: *When things are breaking down.*

The three symptoms that indicate that I am very close to a crisis are:

1.   No longer attending church/participating in spiritual activities
2.   Missing work/school
3.   Increased television

When I notice any of these, I will immediately:

- Seek support from my therapist, psychiatrist/primary care, and other support systems.

CRISIS PLAN

Part 1: *What I'm like when I'm feeling well.*
When I am feeling well, I am committed to my relationship with Christ through my personal devotion as well as through attending church and/or fellowshipping with other Believers. I am committed to my personal goals and in excelling spiritually, emotionally, mentally, physically, intellectually, educationally, professionally, financially, and relationally. I strive to make an impact in the life of others. I devote myself to relationships that are important to me. I am full of life and hopeful about my future.

Part 2: *Symptoms*
Extreme fatigue/exhaustion, anxiousness, brain fogginess, hopelessness, thoughts of death

This may be visible through the following: Messy home, car, and workspace, poor hygiene, missing work/school, not attending church or other spiritual activities, not paying bills or handling other important business, not keeping appointments or other prior commitments, isolating, not communicating with others, deactivation from social media, poor eating habits, weight gain, lack of exercise.

Part 3: *Supporters*
Doctor: (Name and Phone Number)
Psychiatrist: (Name and Phone Number)
Therapist: (Name and Phone Number)

Mark, Brother   (Name and Phone Number)
Michele, Friend   (Name and Phone Number)
Natasha, Friend   (Name and Phone Number)
Kelli, Friend   (Name and Phone Number)

Part 4: *Medication*
(Anti-Depression)
(Allergies)
(Asthma)
(Vitamins)

Part 5: *Treatment*
*I do not wish to use electric shock treatment.

Part 6: *Home/Community Care/Respite Center*
My desire is to receive care at home. If symptoms are not controlled through therapy and medication the next step would be outpatient hospitalization before inpatient.

Part 7: *Treatment Facilities*
I have only been to the Brook Hospital. Although it was not the best care, it is the only care I have received.

*I do not wish to be treated at Our Lady of Peace or Seven Counties.

Part 8: *Help from Others*
Help with contacting work/school if unable to attend, help with contacting supports, including primary care physician/psychiatrist, and therapist, help with cleaning home, car, and work space, help with ensuring that bills are paid, help with providing healthy meals, support in exercising, help with shopping for necessities, help with reaching out for help.

Part 9: *Inactivating the Plan*
I no longer need to use this Crisis Plan when I am in Recovery. (See Wellness Plan.)

I developed this plan on October 26, 2021, independently.

The key thing to realize is that dealing with mental illness is not like having a cold. In most cases, if left untreated, it will not just go away on its own, but it requires lots of attention and support. Deciding to serve as someone else's support as they navigate through their healing process can be one of the greatest gifts that you can ever give and that they can ever receive. A final thing I would like to add is that if you think your loved one is in jeopardy of harming themselves or others, please do not hesitate to seek help. I have called the crisis police department or guided someone else to do so a few times in order to save a life. It is better to be safe than sorry. Try to put yourself in someone else's shoes and consider what you would want them to do for you if you were them. That is all that compassion really is, is doing what Atticus suggests in the classic book, To Kill a Mockingbird, understanding a person by considering things from his point of view. Be the help that you would want to receive and do what my former first lady (former Pastor's wife) Sandra Payton, often says, help like you want to be helped. You may not be able to do everything for them, and you cannot, nor should you try, but you can do something. You can never give up on them. You can stand by their side, and you can walk with them, step by step on their journey out of depression.

POEM

I Stopped and I Started

One day, I just stopped.
Stopped regretting my past.
Stopped worrying about my future.
Stopped forcing relationships.
Stopped attaching myself to toxicity.
Stopped rushing time.
Stopped trying to please others.
Stopped living according to the expectations of others.
Stopped being ashamed of my present state.
Stopped begging for love and attention.
Stopped fighting against my purpose.
Stopped wasting time.
Stopped not making myself a priority.
Stopped wallowing in my challenges.
Stopped trying to save everybody.
Stopped overthinking everything.
Stopped being unhappy.
Stopped living a limited life.
Stopped being silenced about what I believe.
Stopped having doubt.

Stopped feeling disappointed, discouraged, hopeless, and inadequate.
Stopped denying my true feelings and thoughts.
Stopped leading an unhealthy lifestyle.
Stopped living less than my best life.
Stopped comparing myself to others.
Stopped trying to be like others.
Stopped believing the lies.
Stopped stunting my own growth.
Stopped adjusting who I am at my core to accommodate others.
Stopped dimming my own light.
Stopped hiding and not using my gifts.
Stopped being a yes and me too person.
Stopped going along to get along.
Stopped being put in a box.
Stopped being afraid.
Stopped basing my happiness on other people and situations.
Stopped giving second chances where there was no true remorse and change in behavior.
Stopped not having boundaries.
Stopped not doing my part.
Stopped not showing up for me as me for me.
Stopped not holding myself and others accountable.
Stopped self-blaming for things beyond my control.
Stopped taking everything personal.

Stopped not taking things personal.
Stopped not sharing my challenges.
Stopped not sharing my celebrations.
Stopped not sharing my experience and wisdom.
Stopped relying on others.
Stopped saying I can't.
Stopped trying to prove myself.
Stopped hating my body and my features.
Stopped pitying my shortcomings.
Stopped not recognizing my inner and outer beauty.
Stopped devaluing myself.
Stopped denying and hiding my true worth.
Stopped allowing others to misuse and abuse me.
Stopped being weak.
Stopped living beneath my privilege.
One day, I just stopped.
And, I.......I started.

CHAPTER 13

And One To Grow On

Originally, my book was to be released November of 2022. However, I pushed the date back to January of 2023. I had been dealing with a lot of stress from school, and symptoms of depression and anxiety were resurfacing. I thought if I could make it to my winter break, I would have the time and energy to finish editing my book so it could be released in January. Unfortunately, when winter break arrived, I was unable to follow through with my commitment. I only had two weeks off before January Term began. The last week of the Fall Semester I became ill. I went to the urgent care twice and to my doctor. I was treated for an upper respiratory infection and an ear infection. I took antibiotics and steroids (Prednisone) for at least three weeks. It took almost a month before I started feeling better physically. Aside from taking my father to several doctor appointments, I spent most of my winter break in bed. At first, I thought I was in bed because of the infections. Then, I realized it was more than that. I was dealing with depression again. I could not believe it. How did I allow myself to get in this place again? How was I going to release a book about overcoming depression when I had not truly overcome myself? I spoke to my publisher and explained to her what I was experiencing. My original thought was to allow the book to be released without me reviewing it. There was an editor who had edited it and made suggestions for changes. I would simply agree with those changes and move forward to not disappoint those who had already purchased the book during pre-sales. When I talked to Michele about it, she was in agreement. She was aware I was struggling again, and she did not want the book to be another layer of stress for me. However, when I talked to my publisher, she convinced me that I really should review the book before releasing it, that this was my baby and that I would want to make sure I was satisfied with it. She was right. We decided to delay releasing the book once again, only this time, it would be indefinitely. I would not put a date on it to avoid any added pressure. My hope was I would be able to review it during my next big break, which would be during the summer, and that I would not set a release date until I had done so. I felt bad about this decision because I felt I would be disappointing some people, but I knew it was for the best.

During my conversation with my publisher, she said something that was very real and powerful. She said I was living out my book in real time and that I would have to use my book as a tool to help myself in the way I intended for it to help others. She was right again. I remembered reading Gospel artist Mandisa's book, Out of the Dark, and how she shared that she was somewhat hesitant to share her story because she knew that her fight was not over. She did not want to give the impression that overcoming depression was a one-time event or something that you would never have to endure again once you were healed from it. I did not want to give this impression either. I had overcome depression many times before, and even though I had experienced great victory, I knew it would not be the last time I would have to face it. I did not anticipate it resurfacing as soon as it did and as intense as it did, but it did. The MAFT program at the Seminary was extremely overwhelming, and it was this way from the very start at orientation. One of my peers experienced a panic attack during orientation and emergency responders were contacted. In my previous Master's programs, two classes were considered full-time status, whereas here, I was taking four courses. I thought it would not be as stressful because I was no longer working. I had resigned from my teaching position at the end of the summer. My friends even had a surprise "Almost Retirement" party for me which was a tremendous blessing to me. I also thought that the healthy habits I had developed during my time off would help carry me through. Unfortunately, I was not prepared for the anxiety I would experience during my first semester. I was enrolled in a class that was very stressful. My cohort and I found out we technically should not have been in the class, that it was a class for upper-level students. Yet, we had no choice but to take it and to do our best. The amount of reading assigned in this class in particular was beyond overwhelming. Eventually, I learned

I could not read every word but that I had to skim some things. There were a lot of other stressful things that occurred, and I did not handle them very well. Sadly, I abandoned pretty much all of the healthy/self-care habits I had developed during my healing. I was not going to church. I was not maintaining my devotion. I was not consistently taking my medication and vitamins. I was not eating healthy. I was not exercising. I had started isolating again from my family and friends. The only thing I was able to do was my schoolwork, and that was extremely difficult. Many times, throughout the semester I wanted to quit. My therapist was even concerned with the amount of anxiety this program was causing me and whether it was wise for me to pursue it. The good part is that I finished the semester and I earned 2 A's and 2 A-'s; the bad part is that I had done so at the expense of my own mental health. Looking back, I would have much rather earned lower grades and taken better care of myself. I was angry, only I did not know who to direct my anger toward. Was it the school's fault for causing all the unnecessary stress? I was not the only person who was suffering, or was it my fault for allowing myself to become so stressed and filled with anxiety? I was so disappointed with myself. I gained forty of the seventy pounds I had previously lost. I was devastated and ashamed.

Releasing my book was the last thing I wanted to do. I wanted it to be released when I was in a position of strength and victory, not weakness and defeat. Then, I remembered how my publisher had encouraged me to use the tools I shared in my book to help myself. So, I asked myself, what were the things I did the last time to help lift myself out of depression. I realized I would need these tools, not only now, but for any other time I experienced a depressive episode in the future. This was not a one-time battle, but I was determined to have victory however many times I had to fight. As I entered January Term, I committed to using these tools that had proven themselves to be effective. I would do the following:

1. Return to my personal devotion time and to attending church.

2. See my doctor and share with him what I had been experiencing.

3. Be completely honest with my therapist and work on developing better coping skills.

4. Resume taking my medication and vitamins and using my light therapy consistently.

5. Resume my healthy diet.

6. Resume exercising.

7. Work on reconnecting to my family and friends.

8. Make time for fun and enjoyment.

9. Get proper rest.

These tools had worked for me before; therefore, I knew they could work for me again if only I used them. One of the things I have learned about depressive episodes is you cannot always control when they appear, but you can control how long they remain. Now in the last week or so, I have been able to combat the depression, and I have felt much better each day. During the brief time I had off in between January Term and the Spring Semester, I was able to review my book. When I read the last chapter, I realized I wanted to add this final piece to share the challenge I experienced after writing the book. I would have never thought I would have to use my own book to help myself, at least not this soon, but I did, and it worked. Now, I am even more committed to doing what it takes to overcome depression and to maintain my mental health. Anything worth having is worth fighting for, and I intend to keep doing just that. I look forward to sharing more about my journey as I learn and grow in my studies and in my personal experience. Thank you for allowing me to share my journey thus far from the depth of my soul. It has brought me much healing and great joy to know that I have overcome so much already and that I will continue to overcome; for I am more than a conqueror through Him that loves me.

ABOUT THE AUTHOR

Lichelle is a former high school teacher of twenty plus years. She holds a BS in Secondary Education, Speech Communications, Theatre Arts, and English from Ball State University, and a MS in Secondary Education from Indiana University. She has done study in social work at the graduate level through Kent School at the University Louisville. She is now pursuing a MA in Marriage and Family Therapy at Louisville Presbyterian Theological Seminary. It was Lichelle's personal battle with depression that led to her new life purpose and passion.

Lichelle is also a minister of the Gospel. She has been teaching and preaching the Word of God for over twenty years. She has been most effective in helping women overcome life's challenges and to live victoriously. It is her desire to reach as many people as she possibly can through her story. For those who also struggle with depression, she wants them to learn from her experience how they too, can overcome. For those with loved ones who struggle with depression, she wants them to understand the impact it has on their entire life and understand how they can be of greater support. Her mission is to share her story, to stand up for and with others, and to lend support in helping others develop inner peace. Great things are in store for her in her near future. She intends to finish school and have a private practice as well as to continue to write more books and to travel around the world sharing her story and teaching others how to overcome depression as well.

As her focus, she uses the Scripture in which Christ told Peter that once he had been restored to go back and strengthen the brethren. That is what she intends to do, to go back and lead others out of darkness. She is committed to being the help that she wishes she had, and she will strive all the more earnestly to reach her goal.

CPSIA information can be obtained
at www.ICGtesting.com
Printed in the USA
LVHW032336240323
742479LV00002B/295

9 781955 107679